MEAL PREP GUIDE FOR BEGINNERS

Healthy Meal Prep Recipes to Lose Weight and Save Time for Your Family

(Healthy and Wholesome Ketogenic Meals to Prep Grab)

Kerrie Lowe

Published by Alex Howard

© **Kerrie Lowe**

All Rights Reserved

Meal Prep Guide for Beginners: Healthy Meal Prep Recipes to Lose Weight and Save Time for Your Family (Healthy and Wholesome Ketogenic Meals to Prep Grab)

ISBN 978-1-990169-73-1

All rights reserved. No part of this guide may be reproduced in any form without permission in writing from the publisher except in the case of brief quotations embodied in critical articles or reviews.

Legal & Disclaimer

The information contained in this book is not designed to replace or take the place of any form of medicine or professional medical advice. The information in this book has been provided for educational and entertainment purposes only.

The information contained in this book has been compiled from sources deemed reliable, and it is accurate to the best of the Author's knowledge; however, the Author cannot guarantee its accuracy and validity and cannot be held liable for any errors or omissions. Changes are periodically made to this book. You must consult your doctor or get professional medical advice before using any of the suggested remedies, techniques, or information in this book.

Table of contents

Part 1 1
Introduction 2
Italian Sausage and Zucchini 4
Sheet Pan Chicken Fajitas 5
Bodega Bay Cioppino 6
Cabbage and Noodles 8
Crazy-Simple Cottage Ham, Potatoes, and Green Beans 9
Slow Cooker Venison Stroganoff Meal 10
Unstuffed Cabbage Dinne 11
Chicken Tinola 13
Sheet Pan Shrimp Fajitas 14
Asopao de Pollo 15
Deep Fried Corn Meal Sticks with Dipping Sauce 16
One Pan Thai Coconut Yellow Curry Chicken & Rice 18
Chili Maple Lime Salmon Bowls with Forbidden Rice 20
Slow Cooker Black Bean Quinoa Pumpkin Chicken Chili 21
Spicy Thai Peanut Chicken & Sweet Potato Noodle Stir Fry 23
Vegetarian Tofu Cashew Coconut Curry 25
Amazing Slow Cooker Turkey Tacos 26
Golden Turmeric Chickpea Chicken Soup 28
Healthy Slow Cooker Chicken Tikka Masala 29
Spicy Maple Glazed Salmon 31
Slow Cooker Salsa Verde Chicken Chickpea Chili 32
Thai Peanut Chicken, Edamame & Quinoa Stir Fry 33
Butternut Squash, Chickpea & Lentil Moroccan Stew 35

Kung Pao Chickpea & Brussels Sprouts Stir Fry 37

The Best Healthy Turkey Chili 39

Butternut Squash Green Chile Chicken Soup 40

Slow Cooker Taco Lentil Soup 42

Stuffed Poblano Peppers with Black Bean, Corn & Sweet Potato 43

Golden Coconut Chicken Lentil Soup 44

Blackened Salmon Tacos with Forbidden Rice & Mango Guacamole 46

Cranberry Pecan Quinoa Stuffed Acorn Squash with Goat Cheese Crema 47

Healing Lemongrass Chickpea Thai Green Curry 49

Quick & Easy Chicken Spring Roll Jars 52

Honey Sriracha Glazed Meatballs 53

LIGHTENED UP SWEET AND SOUR CHICKEN 55

SMOKEY GREEN BEAN TURKEY SKILLET 56

Spicy Peanut Chicken Wraps 57

Sausage with Summer Squash 58

TACO MEAL PREP BOWLS 60

Loaded Breakfast Stuffed Peppers 61

Greek Quinoa Breakfast Bowl 63

Spinach, Feta and Egg Breakfast Quesadillas 64

Teriyaki Chicken and Broccoli 65

Quinoa Egg Breakfast Muffin Recipe 67

Peanut butter & jam breakfast cookies 68

Healthy Freezer Breakfast Sandwiches 69

Maple Apple Steel Cut Oats 70

Healthy Chicken and Veggies 71

BANANA ZUCCHINI OATMEAL CUPS 72
Strawberry Banana Baked Oatmeal 73
Part 2 75
Introduction 76
Chapter 1: Salad Recipes 77
Flavorful Chef's Salad 77
Buttery Lettuce with Egg and Potato 78
Chicken Salad with Almonds and Green Beans 80
Chicken, Pistachio, and Feta Salad 81
Turkey Taco Salad 82
Spinach Salad with Salmon 83
Steak and Arugula Salad 84
Rice and Black Bean Salad with Chicken 86
Lite Cobb Salad 87
Shrimp and Cucumber Salad 88
Ham, Egg, and Spinach Salad 89
White-bean Shrimp Salad 90
Mediterranean Salad 91
Chicken and Mango Salad 92
Asian Rotisserie Chicken Salad 93
Romaine, Avocado, and Tuna Salad 94
Citrus-Infused Steak Salad 95
Soba Noodle Salad with Chicken 96
Tortilla, Bean, and Corn Salad 97
Tuna, Celery, and Cucumber Salad 98
Chapter 2: Chicken Recipes 100
Grilled Chicken and Roasted Kale 100

Homemade Chicken Fingers ... 102
Marinated Chicken Breasts ... 103
Apple-Honey Drumsticks ... 104
Honey-Mustard Chicken with Apples ... 106
Creamy Lemon-Pepper Orzo with Grilled Chicken ... 108
Middle Eastern Chicken, Veggies, and Rice ... 109
Sesame-Lemon Chicken ... 111
Roasted Rosemary Chicken ... 112
Honey Mustard and Red Onion BBQ Chicken ... 113
Crunchy French Onion Chicken ... 115
3 Ingredient Chicken Breasts ... 116
Fiesta Slow Cooker Shredded Chicken Tacos ... 117
Simple Roasted Chicken ... 118
Pesto Chicken ... 119
Grilled Chicken Skewers ... 120
Chicken Quesadilla ... 122
Coconut-Curry Chicken ... 123
Grilled Chicken and Pineapple Sandwiches ... 124
Vietnamese Stir-Fry ... 126
Slow Cooker Buffalo Chicken Lettuce Wraps ... 127
Chapter 3: Beef and Pork ... 129
Brussel Sprouts and Sausage ... 129
Dijon-Brown Sugar Steak ... 130
Easy 3 Ingredient Chili ... 131
Grilled PB & B&B Sandwich ... 133
Cajun Dijon Grilled Pork Tenderloin ... 134
Mexican Stuffed Peppers ... 135

- Asian Meatballs 136
- Porcupine Meatballs 138
- Stuffed Tomatoes 140
- Mini Meatloaves with Green Beans and Potatoes 141
- Chapter 4: Breakfast Recipes 144
- Brie and Cranberry Phyllo Turnovers 144
- Paleo Pancakes 145
- Chia Pudding 146
- Chocolate Chip Oatmeal Breakfast Cookie 147
- Cheddar Broccoli Egg Muffin 148
- Almond Butter Granola Bars 149
- Flourless Peanut Butter Muffins 150
- Ham, Kale, Cauliflower, and Egg Muffins 151
- Fruit and Yogurt Cups 152
- Breakfast Taquitos 153
- Meal prep recipes 155
- Italian Veggie Salad 156
- Edamame and Soba Noodle Bowl 157
- Cucumber, Lemon, and Sage Sipper 159
- Vegan Lentils with Kale Artichoke Saute 161
- Vegan Taco Appetizers 163
- Veggie-Cashew Stir-Fry 165
- Vibrant Black-Eyed Pea Salad 167
- Quick Taco Wraps 168
- Colorful Spiral Pasta Salad 170
- Avocado Bruschetta 172
- Tomato-Garlic Lentil Bowls 174

Pressure-Cooker Caponata 176
Herb-Vinaigrette Potato Salad 178
Vegetarian Pad Thai 180
Mediterranean Bulgur Salad 182
Veggie Quiche Bundles 184
Lentil Taco Cups 186
Grilled Feta Quesadillas 188
Conclusion 190

Part 1

Introduction

There are different aspects in life that need proper attention and decision making. We've got lots of problems and struggles as we move forward every single day of our lives. The way we handle things together, like balancing them is very important as we see positivity in all things that we are into.

Handling all the life's burden may seem difficult and challenging. We can overcome all these things by simply making a positive outlook that everything will be good at the end of the day.

In the family, the most affected persons in terms of life's challenges are the mothers. They've got busy days, hectic schedules, and different tasks that need to be done. They do the household chores, cook foods, do the laundry, and many more. These things are the reason, mothers are the busiest person in the family.

Some mothers are pre-occupied by all the things that they forgot to maintain their posture, healthy lifestyle and of course a beautiful physique. Because of these, they needed a guide that serve as the solution that monitors the things that mothers need to maintain to live longer and healthier, and that is the complete Meal Prep cookbook.

The complete meal prep cookbook helps everyone, not only mothers but also of all ages that wanted to live a healthier lifestyle. Dreaming and maintaining a healthy lifestyle full of burdens may seem to be impossible to mothers. Because of this, the complete meal prep cookbook is made.

BENEFITS

1.   Suits your budget.

Before going to the grocery store, you need to plan ahead of time. List all the possible goods that your family really needs. The foods that you are going to cook for breakfast, lunch and dinner. This preparation is important so you could not buy the things that are unnecessary and ended into the trash.

2.   Saves your time.

Meal prepping using the complete meal prep cookbook, will minimize your rush take-outs in some fast food chains out there. You will be able to manage your time in going to the gym and doing your fitness goals because the foods that you are going to make are already prepared for you.

3.   You can make varieties of food each week.

The complete meal prep cookbook will help you decide what to eat in every meal. You can try a new recipe after the other since you already have planned and prepared for it.

So, those are the things that you'll get once you will use the complete meal prep cookbook. You will realize that maintaining a healthy lifestyle isn't that hard, challenging may be but a healthy lifestyle begins within yourself. The encouragement that you have within yourself, will bring you into a healthy lifestyle that sooner or later you can maintain. There's no such thing as difficult in healthy living. The fact that you have the determination and endurance every day, then you have the assurance that you will win in every battles in your life.

Italian Sausage and Zucchini

Prep Time: 20 minutes
Cook Time: 25 minutes
Total Time: 45 minutes
Serves: 6

INGREDIENTS
- 1 1/2 lb Italian sausage links
- 2 S zucchini (sliced)
- 1 S yellow squash (sliced)
- 1/2 c chopped onion
- 1 (14.5z) can stewed tomatoes (with liquid)

INSTRUCTIONS

4. In a skillet, add the sausages and cook over medium heat until no longer pink.
5. Cut into ¼" slice and continue to cook until browned.
6. Add the onion, yellow squash, and zucchini and stir for 2 minutes.
7. Add the tomatoes.
8. Reduce the heat to low. Cover and then simmer the mixture for about 15 minutes.

Sheet Pan Chicken Fajitas

Prep Time: 35 minutes
Cook Time: 15 minutes
Total Time: 50 minutes
Serves: 5

INGREDIENTS

- 1/3 c vegetable oil
- 2 tsp chili powder
- 1 tsp dried oregano
- 1/2 tsp garlic powder
- 1/2 tsp onion powder
- 1/2 tsp ground cumin
- 1/2 tsp salt
- 1/4 tsp black pepper
- 1 pinch ground cayenne pepper
- 1 1/2 lb chicken tenders (quartered)

- 4 c sliced bell peppers
- 1 onion (sliced)
- 1/4 c fresh cilantro (chopped)
- 1/2 lime (juiced)

INSTRUCTIONS

1. In a resealable plastic bag, add the cayenne pepper, pepper, salt, cumin, onion, garlic, oregano, chili powder and vegetable oil. Combine these ingredients.
2. Add onion, bell peppers and chicken. Shake the mixture to combine.
3. Put in the refrigerator for about 30 minutes.
4. Preheat the oven to 400°F. Line a rimmed sheet pan, using aluminum foil.
5. Pour chicken into the pan and spread.
6. Roast in the oven for about 15 minutes, stirring halfway.
7. Pour lime juice and sprinkle cilantro. Toss mixture.

Bodega Bay Cioppino

Prep Time: 45 minutes
Cook Time: 90 minutes
Total Time: 135 minutes

Serves: 8

INGREDIENTS
- 2 tbsp olive oil
- 1 L onion (chopped)
- 3 cloves crushed garlic
- 2 (28 oz) cans diced tomatoes (with juice)
- 1/2 c dry white wine
- 1/4 c chopped fresh parsley
- 1/2 tsp dried basil
- 2 tsp salt
- 1/2 tsp cracked black pepper
- 1 bay leaf
- 1 lb scallops
- 24 littleneck clams
- 1 1/2 lb crab legs
- 1 lb large fresh shrimp (unpeeled)

INSTRUCTIONS

1. In a heavy pot, add olive oil over medium-high heat.
2. Add garlic and onion, then cook until soft.
3. Pour the white wine and tomatoes into the mixture. Season with bay leaf, pepper, salt, basil, and parsley. Lower heat to medium-low and then simmer the mixture for an hour.

4. Add shrimp, crab legs, clams, scallops, and clams. Cover and then cook over medium heat until the clams have open.
5. Serve in a bowl.

Cabbage and Noodles

Prep Time: 10 minutes
Cook Time: 35 minutes
Total Time: 45 minutes
Serves: 4

INGREDIENTS
- 1 (8 oz) package egg noodles
- 3 tbsp butter
- 1/2 lb bacon
- 1 onion (chopped)
- 1 S head cabbage (chopped)
- garlic salt

INSTRUCTIONS

1. In a large pot, fill with lightly salted water and bring to a boil over high heat.
2. Add the egg noodles and bring to a boil. Cook noodles uncovered while occasionally stirring for 5 minutes or until firm. Drain.

3. Return the cooked egg noodles to the pot and add butter; stir
4. In a skillet, add the bacon and cook over medium-high heat for 10 minutes. Drain to a plate lined with paper towels.
5. Using the same skillet, add the onions and stir over medium heat for 2 minutes.
6. Add cabbage and cook for 5 minutes.
7. Chop the bacon and add into the skillet cooking for 10 minutes.
8. Add the noodles to the skillet and continue to cook until heated through.

Crazy-Simple Cottage Ham, Potatoes, and Green Beans

Prep Time: 15 minutes
Cook Time: 55 minutes
Total Time: 70 minutes
Serves: 6

INGREDIENTS
- 1 (3 lb) cottage ham
- 4 russet potatoes (peeled and halved lengthwise)
- 3 (14.5 oz) cans cut green beans (drained)
- 1 white onion (sliced thickly)
- water

INSTRUCTIONS

1. Put the ham into the Dutch oven.
2. Surround ham with onion slice, green beans, and potato halves. Cover mixture with water.
3. Cover mixture and boil.
4. Reduce heat to medium-low and simmer for 55 minutes.
5. Remove ham and cut to desired thickness.
6. Serve with the vegetables.

Slow Cooker Venison Stroganoff Meal

Prep Time: 10 minutes
Cook Time: 4 hours and 10 minutes
Total Time: 4 hours and 20 minutes
Serves: 4

INGREDIENTS
- 3 tbsp olive oil
- 1 lb venison stew meat (cubed)
- 1 tsp salt
- 1 tsp ground black pepper
- 1 tsp garlic powder
- 1 tsp onion powder

- 1 tbsp all-purpose flour
- 1 c water
- 1 (10.75 oz) can mushroom soup condensed cream
- 1 (16 oz) package egg noodles (uncooked)

INSTRUCTIONS

1. In a skillet, add olive oil over medium-high heat.
2. Add venison, onion powder, garlic powder, pepper, and salt. Toss the ingredients and cook for 8 minutes.
3. Transfer to a slow cooker, leaving some oil on the skillet.
4. Using the same skillet, reduce heat to medium-low. Add flour, cook and stir for 5 minutes until golden brown.
5. Pour water and simmer. Pour into the slow cooker with the soup. Cover mixture and cook over low mode for 4 hours.
6. In a pot, add lightly salted water and boil. Add noodles and cook for 8 minutes. Drain.
7. Spoon the stroganoff over noodles and serve.

Unstuffed Cabbage Dinne

Prep Time: 30 minutes
Cook Time: 30 minutes

Total Time: 60 minutes
Serves: 4

INGREDIENTS

- 1 lb ground beef
- 3/4 tsp garlic powder
- 1 tsp ground black pepper
- 1 (14.5 oz) can low-sodium beef broth
- 1 (1 oz) envelope dry onion soup mix
- 1/2 S onion (chopped)
- 1 c instant white rice
- 2 c green cabbage (coarsely shredded)
- 1 1/2 c tomato-vegetable juice cocktail

INSTRUCTIONS

1. In a skillet, add ground beef and cook over medium-high heat until crumbled. Add onion and season with pepper and garlic powder. Cook and stir until the ground meat is browned.
2. Drain excess fats.
3. Pour onion soup and beef broth in the skillet. Stir to blend the mixture.
4. Bring to a boil.
5. Add cabbage, vegetable juice, and rice.
6. Stir and cover then simmer for 30 minutes over low heat.

Chicken Tinola

Prep Time: 30 minutes
Cook Time: 25 minutes
Total Time: 55 minutes
Serves: 4

INGREDIENTS
- 1 tbsp cooking oil
- 1 onion (chopped)
- 2 cloves minced garlic
- 1 (1 ½ ") piece fresh ginger (peeled and thinly sliced)
- 1 tbsp fish sauce
- 3 lb chicken thighs and legs (rinsed and patted dry)
- 2 (14 oz) cans chicken broth
- 1 chayote squash (peeled, cut into bite-sized pcs)
- salt and pepper
- 1 head bok choy (chopped)
- 1/2 lb spinach

INSTRUCTIONS

1. In a pot, add oil over medium heat. Add garlic and onion. Cook and stir until fragrant.
2. Add ginger then stir.
3. Add the chicken and cook for 5 minutes.

4. Add chicken the broth and cook for 5 minutes.
5. Add chayote and simmer for 10 minutes.
6. Season with salt and pepper to taste.
7. Add spinach and bok choy then cook for 2 minutes.
8. Serve hot and enjoy!

Sheet Pan Shrimp Fajitas

Prep Time: 20 minutes
Cook Time: 10 minutes
Total Time: 30 minutes
Serves: 8

INGREDIENTS

- 1 (1 oz) package fajita seasoning
- 1 tbsp olive oil
- 1 1/2 lb raw shrimp (peeled, deveined)
- 1 red bell pepper (cut into strips)
- 1 yellow bell pepper (cut into strips)
- 1 red onion (cut into strips)
- 1 jalapeno pepper (cut into rings)

INSTRUCTIONS

1. Preheat the oven to 450°F.
2. In a bowl, add olive oil and fajita seasoning. Mix these ingredients together.

3. Add shrimp and toss.
4. In a single layer, put the shrimp on a baking sheet. Spread the red and yellow bell peppers, jalapeno pepper, and red onion evenly.
5. Roast in the oven for 10 minutes, Transfer the shrimp to a plate.
6. Broil the pepper mixture for 2 minutes. Transfer to a plate with the shrimp.

Asopao de Pollo

Prep Time: 25 minutes
Cook Time: 35 minutes
Total Time: 60 minutes
Serves: 6

INGREDIENTS
- 2 lb chicken thighs (boneless, skinless)
- 1/2 tsp pepper
- 1 serving adobo seasoning (light)
- 3 tbsp olive oil
- 1 green bell pepper (diced)
- 1 red bell pepper (diced)
- 1 medium onion (diced)
- 4 cloves minced garlic
- 2 tbsp tomato paste
- 1 1/2 c medium-grain rice
- 2 (14.5 oz) cans diced tomatoes
- 6 c chicken broth (low-sodium)

- 1 bay leaf
- 1/4 tsp red pepper flakes
- 1 c frozen petite peas (thawed)
- 1 c pimento-stuffed green olives (sliced)
- 1/4 c fresh cilantro (chopped)

INSTRUCTIONS

1. Place the chicken in a medium-sized bowl and season with adobo seasoning and black pepper.
2. In a large pot, add olive oil over medium heat. Add tomato paste, garlic, onion, red pepper, and green pepper; cook and stir for 3 minutes. Transfer the vegetables to a plate and set aside.
3. Using the same pot, add and fry chicken for 5 minutes per side. Return the vegetables. Add red pepper flakes, bay leaf, chicken broth, diced tomatoes, and rice.
4. Bring to a boil and lower the heat to medium-low. Simmer mixture for 20 minutes.
5. Add and stir in olives and peas for 5 minutes.
6. Remove from heat and then discard the bay leaf.
7. Add cilantro and stir. Serve!

Deep Fried Corn Meal Sticks with Dipping Sauce

Prep Time: 30 minutes
Cook Time: 30 minutes
Total Time: 60 minutes
Serves: 6

INGREDIENTS
- 2 c water
- 3 tbsp white sugar
- 1 tbsp butter
- 1 tsp salt
- 1 1/2 c cornmeal
- 3 c vegetable oil for frying
- vegetable oil
- 1/2 c mayonnaise
- 1/4 c ketchup
- 1 pinch garlic salt

INSTRUCTIONS

1. In a saucepan, pour water and bring to a boil. Stir in the salt, butter and sugar. Cook until sugar dissolved.
2. Reduce heat to low and whisk a cup of cornmeal. Cook and stir until smooth then add the remaining cornmeal to make a workable dough.
3. In a saucepan add vegetable oil and heat over 350°F.

4. Scoop 3 tbsp of dough, form into a ball and roll into half-inch wide and 3-inches long.
5. Repeat with the remaining dough.
6. Deep fry until golden brown. Drain on paper towels.
7. In a bowl, mix the salt, ketchup, garlic salt, and mayonnaise.
8. Serve the cornmeal sticks with dipping.

One Pan Thai Coconut Yellow Curry Chicken & Rice

Prep Time: 10 minutes
Cook Time: 30 minutes
Total Time: 40 minutes
Serves: 4

INGREDIENTS
- 1 tbsp coconut oil
- 2 cloves minced garlic
- 1 lb chicken thighs (boneless, skinless)
- salt and pepper
- 2 cloves minced garlic
- 1 tbsp freshly grated ginger
- 1 bunch green onions (chopped)
- 1 red bell pepper (julienned)
- 8 oz green beans (ends trimmed, cut into 2" long pcs)
- 2 M carrots (sliced)

- 1 (15 oz) can lite coconut milk
- 1 tbsp M yellow curry powder
- 1 tsp ground turmeric
- 1 lime (juiced)
- ½ tsp salt
- 1 c white basmati rice

To garnish
- Fresh cilantro
- Diced green onion

INSTRUCTIONS

1. In a skillet, add coconut oil and garlic over medium-high heat.
2. Add the chicken seasoned with salt and pepper. Cook for 5 minutes and flip, then cook for another 5 minutes. Transfer to a plate.
3. Reduce heat to medium. Using the same skillet, add garlic, green beans, ginger, carrots, red bell pepper and green onion. Saute for 4 minutes.
4. Add salt, lime juice, turmeric, curry powder, and coconut milk then stir to combine. Simmer and fold in the rice.
5. Add chicken on top and reduce heat to low. Cover skillet and cook for 20 minutes.
6. Garnish with green onion and cilantro.

Chili Maple Lime Salmon Bowls with Forbidden Rice

Prep Time: 5 minutes
Cook Time: 25 minutes
Total Time: 30 minutes
Serves: 2

INGREDIENTS
- 2 (6 ounces) wild salmon filets
- 1 tbsp pure maple syrup
- 1 S lime (juiced)
- 1 tsp chili powder
- 3 cloves minced garlic
- 1 tsp virgin coconut oil
- 1/2 c black rice (uncooked)
- 1/2 mango (diced)
- 1/2 c cooked shelled edamame
- 1/8 tsp salt

To garnish
- Cilantro and green onion
- Avocado slices

INSTRUCTIONS

1. In a small pot, add rice and a cup of water then let it boil over high heat. Lower the heat to low and cook for about 25 minutes.
2. Stir in, salt, edamame, coconut oil, and mango.
3. Preheat the oven to 400°F. Line baking sheet with parchment papers. Place salmon 2 inches with skin side down.
4. In a bowl, add garlic, chili powder, lime juice, and maple syrup. Whisk these ingredients together. Brush mixture over salmon.
5. Bake for 15 minutes.
6. Put rice mixture in bowls and top with salmon.
7. Garnish with green onion and cilantro.

Slow Cooker Black Bean Quinoa Pumpkin Chicken Chili

Prep Time: 10 minutes
Cook Time: 2 hours and 5 minutes
Total Time: 2 hours and 15 minutes
Serves: 6

INGREDIENTS
- ½ tbsp olive oil
- 3 cloves minced garlic
- 1 white onion (roughly chopped)
- 1 red bell pepper (julienned)

- 1 jalapeño (seeded, diced)
- 1 (28 oz) can crushed tomatoes
- 1 1/2 c water
- 1 (15 oz) can pumpkin puree
- 1 (15 oz) can black beans
- ½ c uncooked quinoa
- ¾ tsp salt
- 2 tbsp chili powder
- 2 tsp cumin
- ¼ tsp cayenne pepper
- 1 lb chicken thighs/breasts (boneless skinless)

INSTRUCTIONS

1. In a pot, add oil over medium-high heat.
2. Add garlic, red bell pepper, onion, and jalapeno. Saute and stir for about 2 minutes; transfer to a slow cooker.
3. Add the water, cayenne pepper, cumin, chili powder, quinoa salt, black beans, pumpkin puree and crushed tomatoes into the slow cooker. Stir well and add the chicken. Cover and cook over high for 2 hours
4. Remove chicken and shred then return to the slow cooker.
5. Do a meal prep.

Spicy Thai Peanut Chicken & Sweet Potato Noodle Stir Fry

Prep Time: 10 minutes
Cook Time: 20 minutes
Total Time: 30 minutes
Serves: 4

INGREDIENTS

For the sauce
- 1/4 c peanut butter
- 2 tbsp soy sauce
- 1/2 tsp ground ginger
- 1 clove finely minced garlic
- 1 tbsp sriracha sauce
- 1/2 tbsp honey
- 1 tsp sesame oil
- 3/4 c unsweetened almond

For the stir fry
- 3 M sweet potatoes (peeled)
- 1 tbsp sesame oil (divided)
- 1 lb chicken breasts (boneless skinless, cut into 1" pcs)
- 2 1/2 c broccoli florets
- 1 L red bell pepper (cut into thin strips)

For garnish
- green onions
- chopped peanuts
  - cilantro

INSTRUCTIONS

1. In a bowl, add almond milk, sesame oil, honey, sriracha, garlic,ginger, soy sauce, and peanut butter. Whisk these ingredients together to make a sauce.
2. Use a spiralizer to your sweet potatoes and make noodles. Set aside
3. Season the chicken to taste with salt and pepper.
4. In a skillet add olive oil over medium-high heat. Add chicken and cook for 6 minutes. Transfer chicken to a plate.
5. Using the same skillet, add sesame oil, broccoli and red pepper flakes. Stir-fry for 2 minutes and add the sweet potato noodles. Then cook for another 2 minutes.
6. Add chicken and peanut sauce. Stir to coat the veggies.
7. Lower heat to medium-low and cook for a few minutes more until noodles are al-dente.
8. Garnish with cilantro, chopped peanuts band green onions.

Vegetarian Tofu Cashew Coconut Curry

Prep Time: 15 minutes
Cook Time: 30 minutes
Total Time: 45 minutes
Serves: 4

INGREDIENTS
- 1 tbsp virgin coconut oil
- 3 cloves minced garlic
- 1 tbsp freshly grated ginger
- 1 jalapeño (diced)
- 1 M sweet potato (diced into 1" cubes)
- ½ head of cauliflower (cut into small florets)
- 1 bell yellow or orange pepper, diced
- 2 carrots (chopped)
- 2 tbsp curry powder
- ½ tsp turmeric
- ½ tsp cumin
- ⅛ tsp ground cinnamon
- ½ tsp salt
- 1 (15 oz) can lite coconut milk
- 1/2 c tomato sauce
- ½ c vegetarian broth
- ¼ c roasted cashews, ground
- 1 package firm Nasoya tofu (cubed)
- Cilantro (to garnish)

INSTRUCTIONS

1. In a large pot, add coconut oil over medium-high heat.
2. Add the carrots, bell pepper, cauliflower, sweet potato, jalapeno, ginger, and garlic, then saute for 10 minutes.
3. Add salt, cinnamon, cumin, turmeric and curry powder, then stir. Add cashews, broth, tomato sauce and coconut milk. Stir mixture until smooth.
4. Add tofu and stir.
5. Turn the heat to low and simmer for about 20 minutes.
6. Serve with cilantro.

Amazing Slow Cooker Turkey Tacos

Prep Time: 10 minutes
Cook Time: 2 hours and 10 minutes
Total Time: 2 hours and 20 minutes
Serves: 4

INGREDIENTS

For the taco meat
- 1 tsp olive oil
- 1 white onion (chopped)
- 1 lb 94% lean ground turkey

- 3 cloves minced garlic
- 1 (8 ounces) can tomato sauce
- 2 tsp cumin
- 2 tsp chili powder
- 1 tsp dried oregano
- ½ tsp paprika
- ⅛ tsp cayenne pepper
- ¾ tsp salt

Toppings
- 8 corn tortillas
- 1 c grape tomatoes (quartered)
- ½ c shredded cheddar cheese
- 1 avocado (diced)
- Shredded lettuce (topping)
- Sliced jalapeno (topping)

INSTRUCTIONS

1. In a skillet, add oil and place over medium-high heat.
2. Add turkey and onion.
3. Break up turkey meat until browned.
4. Transfer to a slow cooker and add salt, cayenne pepper, paprika, oregano, chili powder, cumin, tomato sauce, and garlic. Stir the mixture to combine.
5. Cook on high for 3 hours.

6. Divide meat with 8 tortillas.
7. Add jalapeno, lettuce, avocado, cheese and grape tomatoes.

Golden Turmeric Chickpea Chicken Soup

Prep Time: 10 minutes
Cook Time: 40 minutes
Total Time: 50 minutes
Serves: 4

INGREDIENTS
- 1 tsp coconut oil
- 3 cloves minced garlic
- 2 tsp fresh grated ginger
- 2 jalapenos (seeded and diced)
- 1 lb chicken breast (boneless, skinless, cut into bite size)
- 1 S white onion (diced)
- 1 red pepper (thinly sliced)
- 1 M sweet potato (peeled, diced into small cubes)
- 1 1/4 tsp ground turmeric
- 4 c chicken broth (low sodium)
- 1 (15 ounces) can chickpeas (rinsed, drained)
- 1/2 tsp salt
- black pepper
- 1 c light coconut milk
- 2 tbsp peanut butter (all natural creamy)
- green onions (to garnish)

- Fresh cilantro (to garnish)

INSTRUCTIONS

1. In a pot add, coconut oil over medium-high heat.
2. Add ginger, garlic, chicken breast and jalapeno. Cook and stir for 4 minutes.
3. Add sweet potato, red pepper, and onion. Cook and stir for 5 minutes.
4. Add turmeric and stir to coat.
5. Add salt and pepper, coconut milk, peanut butter, chickpeas, and broth. Stir and bring to a boil.
6. Turn the heat to low and then simmer for 20 minutes, uncovered.
7. Serve in a bowl and top with green onions and cilantro.

Healthy Slow Cooker Chicken Tikka Masala

Prep Time: 10 minutes
Cook Time: 2 hours 25
Total Time: 2 hours 35 minutes
Serves: 4

INGREDIENTS

- 2 tsp olive oil
- 1 S onion (diced)
- 1 jalapeno (seeds removed, finely diced)
- 3 cloves minced garlic
- 1 tbsp fresh grated ginger
- 1 jar (24.5 ounces) Mutti tomato puree
- 1 tbsp fresh lemon juice
- 1 tbsp garam masala
- 1 tsp paprika
- 1/2 tsp cayenne pepper
- 1/2 tsp ground turmeric
- 1/2 tsp curry powder
- black pepper
- 1/4 teaspoon salt
- 1 lb chicken breasts (boneless, skinless)
- 3/4 c light coconut milk
- greek yogurt (garnish)
- Chopped cilantro (garnish)

INSTRUCTIONS

1. In a skillet, add olive oil over medium heat.
2. Add garlic, onion, and jalapeno, then saute for 5 minutes.
3. Transfer to a slow cooker then add curry powder, turmeric, cayenne pepper, paprika, garam masala, lemon juice, and tomato puree. Stir to combine.

4. Add chicken and combine.
5. Cover and cook for about 2 hours on high.
6. Removed chicken to a cutting board and shred with forks.
7. Return to the slow cooker then add coconut milk. Cook on high for 15 minutes uncovered.
8. Garnish with yogurt and cilantro.

Spicy Maple Glazed Salmon

Prep Time: 5 minutes
Cook Time: 20 minutes
Total Time: 25 minutes
Serves: 2

INGREDIENTS
- 2 (6 oz each) wild salmon filets
- 1 tbsp pure maple syrup
- 1 tbsp reduced sodium soy sauce
- 1 tsp dijon mustard
- 1 tsp chili powder
- 1/4 tsp cayenne pepper
- 1 garlic minced clove

INSTRUCTIONS

1. Preheat the oven to 350°F. And line a baking sheet with parchment papers.
2. Place fish fillets 2" apart on baking sheet.
3. In a bowl, add garlic, cayenne pepper, chili powder, dijon mustard, soy sauce and maple syrup. Whisk these ingredients together.
4. Brush over the fish fillets and reserve 2 tbsp.
5. Bake for 20 minutes.
6. Remove from oven and top with the reserved glaze.

Slow Cooker Salsa Verde Chicken Chickpea Chili

Prep Time: 5 minutes
Cook Time: 3 hours
Total Time: 3 hours 5 minutes
Serves: 6

INGREDIENTS

- 2 lb chicken thighs (boneless, skinless)
- 24 ounces mild salsa verde
- 1 onion (chopped)
- 1/2 jalapeno (seeded, diced)
- 2 cloves minced garlic
- 1 c frozen corn
- 1 (15 ounces) can chickpeas
- 1/2 c uncooked quinoa
- 2 1/2 c chicken broth (low sodium)
- 2 small limes (juiced)

- 2 tsp ground cumin
- 2 tsp dried oregano
- Salt and pepper
- Fresh cilantro (garnish)
- Avocado (garnish)
- Tortilla chips (garnish)
- Greek yogurt (garnish)

INSTRUCTIONS

1. IN a slow-cooker, add all the ingredients and stir to combine.
2. Cook for 3 hours on high.
3. Transfer the chicken to a cutting board and then shred with forks then return to slow cooker.
4. Garnish with greek yogurt, tortilla chips, avocado, and cilantro.

Thai Peanut Chicken, Edamame & Quinoa Stir Fry

Prep Time: 10 minutes
Cook Time: 30 minutes
Total Time: 40 minutes
Serves: 4

INGREDIENTS

For the quinoa
- 1/3 c uncooked quinoa
- 2/3 c water

For the sauce
- 1/3 c powdered peanut butter
- 1/4 c almond milk (unsweetened)
- 2 tbsp soy sauce (gluten-free)
- 1/2 tbsp honey
- 1 tsp red wine vinegar
- 3 cloves minced garlic
- 1/4 tsp cayenne pepper

For the stir fry
- 1 tbsp sesame oil (divided)
- 1 lb chicken breast (boneless, skinless, cut into 1" cubes)
- salt and pepper
- 3 c fresh broccoli florets
- 1 M red bell pepper (thinly sliced)
- 1 c frozen organic edamame

For garnish
- roasted peanuts (crushed)
- fresh cilantro
- hot sauce

INSTRUCTIONS

1. Too cook the quinoa, add water and quinoa to a pot and cook over high heat. Bring to a boil and turn the heat to low, then simmer for 15 minutes. Remove from heat and fluff with a fork then set aside.
2. In a bowl, add garlic, vinegar, honey, soy sauce, almond milk, and peanut butter. Whisk until smooth and set aside.
3. Season the chicken with salt and pepper.
4. In a skillet add a half tablespoon of sesame oil over medium-high heat.
5. Add chicken and cook for 6 minutes. Transfer chicken to a plate,
6. Using the same skillet add another half tablespoon of sesame oil. Add edamame, red pepper slices, and broccoli florets. Stir-fry for 6 minutes and season with salt and pepper.
7. Return the chicken and add the peanut sauce then stir.
8. Reduce heat to medium-low and add quinoa. Stir the mixture,
9. Garnish with hot sauce, peanuts, and cilantro.

Butternut Squash, Chickpea & Lentil Moroccan Stew

Prep Time: 15 minutes
Cook Time: 30 minutes
Total Time: 45 minutes
Serves: 4

INGREDIENTS

- 1 tsp olive
- 1 white onion (chopped)
- 6 cloves garlic (crushed)
- 2 tsp cumin
- 1/2 tsp cinnamon
- salt and pepper
- 1 can (15 ounces) chickpeas (rinsed, drained)
- 1 can (28 ounces) diced tomatoes
- 3 c vegetable broth (organic)
- 1 lb butternut squash (diced large)
- 1 c green lentils (rinsed well)
- 1/8 tsp saffron
- 1/2 lemon (juiced)
- red pepper flakes (few dashes)
- 1/3 c cilantro (chopped) plus more for garnish
- basil leaf (chopped)
- Greek yogurt (for garnish)

INSTRUCTIONS

1. In a pot, add oil over medium heat.
2. Add garlic, and onion then cook until onion softened.
3. Add cinnamon, cumin, and salt and pepper. Cook and stir until fragrant.
4. Add saffron, lentils, butternut squash, broth, tomatoes, and chickpeas.

5. Bring to boil and turn the heat to low.
6. Cover and simmer for 15 minutes.
7. Add basil, cilantro, red pepper flakes and lemon juice; stir.
8. Garnish with cilantro and greek yogurt.

Kung Pao Chickpea & Brussels Sprouts Stir Fry

Prep Time: 10 minutes
Cook Time: 15 minutes
Total Time: 25 minutes
Serves: 4

INGREDIENTS

For the stir fry
- 2 tbsp sesame oil
- 1 lb brussels sprouts (halved)
- salt and pepper
- 1 red onion (chopped)
- 1 red bell pepper (chopped)
- 1 (15 oz) can chickpeas (rinsed, drained)

For the kung pao sauce
- 3 garlic minced cloves
- 1 tsp red pepper flakes
- 1 tsp freshly grated ginger
- 1 tbsp apple cider vinegar
- 2 tbsp gluten-free soy sauce
- 1 tsp coconut sugar

- ½ tbsp cornstarch
- 2 tbsp peanut butter

To garnish:
- Red pepper flakes
- Chopped peanuts
- Green onions
- Cilantro

INSTRUCTIONS

1. To make the kung pao sauce, in a bowl add the peanut butter, cornstarch, coconut sugar, soy sauce, cider vinegar, ginger red pepper flakes, and garlic. Whisk ingredients until the cornstarch then set aside.
2. In a skillet, add sesame oil over medium-high heat. Add the Brussel sprouts and then cook for about 3 minutes.
3. Add red bell pepper and red onion, then saute for another 3 minutes.
4. Add salt and pepper and chickpeas.
5. Reduce heat to low and pour kung pao sauce into the skillet.
6. Stir for 2 minutes. Serve over brown rice or quinoa.
7. Garnish with red pepper flakes, cilantro, green onion, and peanuts.

The Best Healthy Turkey Chili

Prep Time: 10 minutes
Cook Time: 45 minutes
Total Time: 55 minutes
Serves: 6

INGREDIENTS
- 2 tsp olive oil
- 1 yellow onion (chopped)
- 3 garlic minced cloves
- 1 M red bell pepper (chopped)
- 1 lb 99% extra lean ground turkey
- 4 tbsp chili powder
- 2 tsp ground cumin
- 1 tsp dried oregano
- 1/4 tsp cayenne pepper
- 1/2 tsp salt
- 1 (28 ounces) can diced tomatoes
- 1 1/4 c chicken broth
- 2 (15 ounces) cans kidney beans, dark red (rinsed, drained)
- 1 (15 ounces) can sweet corn (rinsed, drained)

For topping
- Cheese
- Avocado
- tortilla chips
- Cilantro
- sour cream

INSTRUCTIONS

1. In a pot, add oil over medium-high heat.
2. Add red pepper, garlic, and onion, then saute for 5 minutes.
3. Add ground turkey and cook by breaking up until browned.
4. Add salt, cayenne pepper, oregano, cumin and chili powder. Stir for 20 seconds.
5. Add corn, kidney beans, broth, and tomatoes.
6. Bring to a boil and lower the heat to medium-low. Simmer for half an hour.
7. Garnish with tortilla chips, cilantro, cheese and sour cream.

Butternut Squash Green Chile Chicken Soup

Prep Time: 10 minutes
Cook Time: 30 minutes
Total Time: 40 minutes
Serves: 4

INGREDIENTS

- ½ tbsp olive oil
- 6 cloves minced garlic
- 1 L white onion (chopped)
- 1 green bell pepper (diced small)
- ¼ c diced cilantro

- 1 (4 oz) can chilies (mild green)
- 6 c butternut squash (cubed)
- 1 1/2 tsp ground cumin
- 1 tsp oregano
- 4 c (32 oz) chicken broth
- 1 pound chicken thighs (boneless, skinless)
- 1 (15 oz) can organic corn (drained)
- 1 S lime (juiced)
- ½ tsp salt
- pepper

INSTRUCTIONS

1. In a pot, add oil over medium-high heat.
2. Add cilantro, green pepper, onion, and garlic. Cook until onion is translucent.
3. Add oregano, cumin, butternut squash and green chiles.
4. Cook for a few minutes and add lime juice, salt and pepper, corn, chicken and chicken broth.
5. Bring to a boil and cover. Lower the heat to medium-low and then simmer for 20 minutes.
6. Transfer chicken to a cutting board and shred with forks.
7. Return to the pot, taste and then adjust the seasonings.

Slow Cooker Taco Lentil Soup

Prep Time: 10 minutes
Cook Time: 3 hours
Total Time: 3 hours 10 minutes
Serves: 4

INGREDIENTS

- 4 cloves minced garlic
- 1 red bell pepper (thinly sliced)
- 1 white onion (diced)
- 1 jalapeño (seeded, diced)
- 1 c brown lentils (rinsed)
- 1 (28 ounces) can crushed tomatoes
- 4 c vegetarian broth
- 1 (15 oz) can black beans (rinsed, drained)
- 2 tbsp chili powder
- 1 tbsp cumin
- 1 tsp dried oregano
- 1/2 tsp paprika
- 1/4 tsp onion powder
- 1/2 tsp cayenne pepper
- 1 tsp salt
- pepper
- 1 c frozen organic corn

For topping
- 1/2 c Cheddar Shreds

To garnish

- Diced cilantro
- sliced jalapeno
- tortilla chips

INSTRUCTIONS

1. In a skillet, add olive oil over medium-high heat.
2. Add jalapeno, onion, bell pepper and garlic, then saute for 5 minutes. Transfer to the slow cooker.
3. Add all the remaining ingredients except the corn. Stir ingredients and cook for 3 hours on high.
4. 20 minutes before serving, add the corn.
5. Serve into bowls, and top with cheese then garnish with tortilla chips, cilantro, and jalapeno.

Stuffed Poblano Peppers with Black Bean, Corn & Sweet Potato

Prep Time: 15 minutes
Cook Time: 45 minutes
Total Time: 60 minutes
Serves: 10

INGREDIENTS

- 5 L poblano peppers (cut lengthwise)
- 1 (15 ounces) can sweet corn (rinsed, drained)
- 1 (15 ounces) can black beans (rinsed, drained)

- 1/2 c yellow onion (diced)
- 1 S sweet potato (microwaved for 4 minutes and cut into small cubes)
- 1 1/4 c chunky tomato salsa
- 2 tsp chili powder
- 1 tsp cumin
- 1 tsp dried oregano
- 1 cup shredded Cheese
- 1/4 c chopped cilantro (for garnish)

INSTRUCTIONS

1. Preheat the oven to 350°F.
2. Place poblano pepper in a pan.
3. Divide the oregano, cumin, chili powder, tomato salsa, sweet potato, onion, corn and blacks beans evenly into each half of poblano pepper.
4. Cover pan with aluminum foil.
5. Bake for 40 minutes.
6. Remove foil and sprinkle cheese on top.
7. Bake for another 5 minutes and sprinkle with cilantro.
8. Serve with salsa and guacamole.

Golden Coconut Chicken Lentil Soup

Prep Time: 15 minutes
Cook Time: 45 minutes

Total Time: 60 minutes
Serves: 4

INGREDIENTS

- 2 tsp olive oil
- 3 cloves minced garlic
- 1 S white onion (roughly chopped)
- 2 L carrots (sliced)
- 3/4 tsp ground turmeric
- 1 tbsp freshly grated ginger
- 1/2 tsp cumin
- 1/8 tsp cayenne pepper,
- 3 c chicken broth
- 1 (15 ounces) can light coconut milk
- 1 c brown lentils (rinsed)
- 2 c shredded chicken breast
- 1/2 tsp salt
- pepper

For garnish

- fresh chopped cilantro
- extra coconut milk

INSTRUCTIONS

1. In a pot, add olive oil over medium-high heat.
2. Add carrots, onion, and garlic then saute for 5 minutes.
3. Add cayenne pepper, cumin, ginger, and turmeric. Cook for half a minute.

4. Add salt and pepper, shredded chicken, lentils, coconut milk, and chicken broth.
5. Bring to a boil and turn the heat to medium-low. Simmer for 45 minutes uncovered.
6. Pour into bowls and garnish with coconut milk and cilantro.

Blackened Salmon Tacos with Forbidden Rice & Mango Guacamole

Prep Time: 10 minutes
Cook Time: 40 minutes
Total Time: 50 minutes
Serves: 4

INGREDIENTS
- 3/4 c uncooked black rice
- 1 lb fresh salmon
- 1 tbsp blackening seasoning

For guacamole
- 1 M ripe avocado (mashed)
- 1/4 c diced red onion
- 1/2 jalapeno (seeded, minced)
- 1/4 c fresh chopped cilantro
- 1 ripe mango (diced)
- 1 S lime (Zest, juice)
- Salt and pepper

- 8 corn tortillas
- extra cilantro (garnish)
- diced red onion (garnish)

INSTRUCTIONS

1. Cooked rice according to package directions,
2. Preheat the oven to 400°F. Line a baking sheet with parchment papers and grease with olive oil.
3. Place salmon and sprinkle with blackening seasoning.
4. Bake for 15 minutes.
5. In a bowl, add avocado, mango, lime zest and juice, cilantro, jalapeno and red onion. Add salt and pepper then stir to combine and set aside.
6. Flake salmon with fork and discard skin.
7. Add rice and salmon to corn tortillas. Top with a tablespoon of guacamole.

Cranberry Pecan Quinoa Stuffed Acorn Squash with Goat Cheese Crema

Prep Time: 20 minutes
Cook Time: 60 minutes
Total Time: 80 minutes
Serves: 4

INGREDIENTS

For the acorn squash

- 2 M acorn squash (cut in half, seeds removed)
- 4 tsp virgin melted coconut oil
- 2 tbsp brown sugar
- Cinnamon

For the quinoa
- ½ c uncooked quinoa
- 1 ¼ c water
- 2 sprigs thyme leaves
- 1 tsp virgin coconut oil
- 1/2 c freshly squeezed orange juice
- 1/2 tsp honey
- 1/4 tsp turmeric
- 1/4 tsp salt
- 1/2 c dried cranberries
- 1/2 c pecan halves

For the goat cheese crema
- 2 oz goat cheese crumbles
- 1 tsp honey
- 1/2 tsp apple cider vinegar
- 3 tbsp water

INSTRUCTIONS
1. Preheat the oven to 350°F. Line baking sheet with parchment papers.
2. Rub a teaspoon of coconut oil and half tablespoon of brown sugar to each half squash.
3. Sprinkle half squash with cinnamon. Bake for 45 minutes, flesh side down.

4. To make quinoa, add thyme leaves, quinoa, and water to a pot. Bring to a boil, cover and turn the heat to low, simmer for 15 minutes. Fluff with fork.
5. Add turmeric, honey, orange juice, and coconut oil. Stir to combine then fold in the pecans and cranberries.
6. Stuff squash with quinoa mixture and bake for 10 minutes more.
7. To make the drizzle, in a blender add water, cider vinegar, honey, and goat cheese. Blend until creamy.
8. Drizzle each squash and serve

Healing Lemongrass Chickpea Thai Green Curry

Prep Time: 15 minutes
Cook Time: 45 minutes
Total Time: 60 minutes
Serves: **4**

INGREDIENTS:
For the brown rice:
- 1 tsp coconut oil
- 1 c uncooked brown rice

For the Thai green curry:
- 2 tsp olive oil
- 3 cloves minced garlic
- 1/2 L white onion (diced)

- 2 stalks (minced) lemongrass
- 1 cup carrots (diced)
- 1 tbsp freshly minced ginger
- 1 tbsp finely diced fresh basil
- 1 tbsp green curry paste
- 1/2 tsp turmeric
- 1 (15 ounces) can lite coconut milk
- 1/2 c vegetarian broth
- 1 (15 ounces) can chickpeas (rinsed, drained)
- 1 tbsp soy sauce (gluten-free)
- 1 lime (juiced)
- 1/4 tsp salt
- 1 red bell pepper (thinly sliced)
- 1 c frozen peas

To garnish:
- Cilantro
- hot sauce

INSTRUCTIONS:

1. To cook the brown rice, in a pan add brown rice and coconut oil. Toast for 5 minutes over medium heat. Add two and a half cups of water then bring to a boil. Lower heat to low, cover the pot and simmer for 45 minutes.
2. In a separate pot, add the olive oil place over medium-high heat. Add basil, ginger, carrots, lemongrass, onion, and garlic then stir-fry for 5 minutes.

3. Add turmeric and turmeric paste then stir for 30 seconds.
4. Add red bell pepper, salt, lime juice, soy sauce, chickpeas, broth and coconut milk. Stir to combine and bring to a boil.
5. Lower heat to medium-low and simmer for 20 minutes, uncovered.
6. Stir in the frozen peas.
7. Serve in a bowl over brown rice and garnish with cilantro and hot sauce.

Quick & Easy Chicken Spring Roll Jars

Prep Time: 15 minutes
Cook Time: 15 minutes
Total Time: 30 minutes
Serves: 4

INGREDIENTS:

- 1 tablespoon sesame oil
- 1 pound ground chicken
- 2 tablespoon soy sauce
- 2 cloves minced garlic
- 1 tablespoon minced ginger
- 1 bag coleslaw
- 2 teaspoon soy sauce
- 2 cups cooked vermicelli noodles
- 1 cup cucumber (cut into matchsticks)
- 1/2 cup sweet chili sauce
- 1 cup red pepper (sliced)
- 1/3 cup cilantro (chopped)
- 1/4 cup sesame seeds

INSTRUCTIONS

1. In a skillet, add sesame oil place over medium-high heat.

2. Add ground chicken and 2 tablespoons of soy sauce then cook for 2 minutes.
3. Add ginger and garlic then sauter for 7 minutes.
4. Transfer chicken to a plate.
5. Add coleslaw to the pan and 2 teaspoons of soy sauce then saute for 2 minutes.
6. Cook vermicelli noodles according to mfg. Directions.
7. In the mason jars, add the chili sauce to each.
8. Divide chicken, red pepper, cucumber, and coleslaw among jars.
9. Top with sesame seeds, herbs, and vermicelli noodles.
10. Can keep on the fridge for 5 days.

Honey Sriracha Glazed Meatballs

Prep Time: 10 minutes
Cook Time: 30 minutes
Total Time: 40 minutes
Serves: 8

INGREDIENTS
For the meatballs:
- 2 pounds lean ground turkey
- 1 c panko breadcrumbs (whole wheat)
- 2 eggs
- ¼ cup green onions (chopped)
- ½ teaspoon garlic powder

- ½ teaspoon salt
- ½ teaspoon black pepper

For the sauce:
- ¼ cup Sriracha
- 3 tablespoon soy sauce (reduced-sodium)
- 3 tablespoon rice vinegar
- 3 tablespoon honey
- tablespoon grated fresh ginger
- cloves minced garlic
- ½ teaspoon toasted sesame oil

INSTRUCTIONS:

1. Preheat the oven to 375°F.
2. In a bowl, add salt and pepper, garlic powder, green onions, eggs, breadcrumbs, and turkey. Mix until combined. Form mixture into balls, about one and a half-inch in size.
3. Spray baking sheets with cooking spray and place the balls.
4. Bake for 20 minutes.
5. For the sauce, in a saucepan mix all the ingredients and bring to a boil over medium heat. Lower the heat to low and simmer for about 10 minutes.
6. Toss sauce with the meatballs.
7. Serve over brown rice. T
8. op with sesame seeds and green onions.

LIGHTENED UP SWEET AND SOUR CHICKEN

Prep Time: 10 minutes
Cook Time: 20 minutes
Total Time: 30 minutes
Serves: 6

INGREDIENTS:
- 2 tablespoon coconut oil (divided)
- 3 chicken breasts (diced)
- ½ green pepper (diced)
- ½ red pepper (diced)
- ½ pineapple (diced)
- 2 carrots (sliced)
- ½ L yellow onion (sliced)
- 1 teaspoon minced garlic
- 1 cup orange juice
- 2 tablespoon white vinegar
- ¼ cup soy sauce
- ¼ cup chicken broth
- 3 tablespoon honey
- 2 tablespoon water
- 2 tablespoon cornstarch

INSTRUCTIONS:

1. In a skillet, add a tablespoon of coconut oil and place over medium heat.
2. Add chicken and cook through. Transfer chicken to a bowl.
3. Add remaining coconut oil to the skillet, add the minced garlic, pineapple, carrots and bell peppers. Stir, cover and cook for 10 minutes.
4. To make a sauce, in a saucepan add honey, chicken broth, soy sauce, vinegar and orange juice. Bring to a boil. Reduce heat to medium-low and simmer.
5. In a bowl, whisk cornstarch and cold water to make a slurry mixture.
6. Add cornstarch mixture to the sauce then whisk together to combine.
7. Simmer for 2 minutes.
8. Pour the chicken and veggies to the saucepan with sauce.
9. Serve with rice.

SMOKEY GREEN BEAN TURKEY SKILLET

Prep Time: 5 minutes
Cook Time: 15 minutes
Total Time: 20 minutes
Serves: 4

INGREDIENTS:

- 1 tbsp olive oil
- 1 lb lean ground turkey
- 1/2 tsp garlic, minced
- 1 red bell pepper (diced)
- 1/2 yellow onion (diced)
- 2 c fresh green beans (ends removed, cut into 1" length)
- 2 tsp smoke seasoning blend
- 3/4 c chipotle salsa
- pinch of salt

INSTRUCTIONS:

1. In a skillet, add olive oil and place over medium-high heat. Add ground beef and a pinch of salt then cook by breaking for 5 minutes. Remove excess fats.
2. Add garlic, green beans, onion and red pepper. Mix and saute for 3 minutes.
3. Add salsa and seasoning. Mix all the ingredients and thoroughly combine. Turn the heat to low and simmer for 6 minutes.
4. Serve over pasta, rice or quinoa.

Spicy Peanut Chicken Wraps

Prep Time: 5 minutes
Cook Time: 15 minutes

Total Time: 20 minutes
Serves: 4

INGREDIENTS:
2 chicken breasts (diced)
- salt
- pepper

For the spicy peanut sauce
1/2 c peanut butter
2 tbsp tamari
1 tbsp olive oil
2 cloves minced garlic
2 tbsp Sriracha sauce
1 tbsp fresh lime juice
1/4 c water

To assemble
1 package Mann's Broccoli Slaw
1 package tortillas
sliced fruit

INSTRUCTIONS:

1. Heat the pan and add chicken. Season with salt and pepper then cook until heat through.
2. In a bowl, add water, lime juice, sriracha. Garlic, olive oil, tamari, and peanut butter. Mix until thick.
3. Spread butter over tortilla and top with broccoli slaw then put the chicken.

Sausage with Summer Squash

Prep Time: 5 minutes
Cook Time: 10 minutes
Total Time: 15 minutes
Serves: 8

INGREDIENTS:
- 4 pork sausage, mild
- 2 plum tomatoes, quartered
- 1 lb zucchini and squash slices
- 1/3 cup Kalamata olives, sliced
- 2 tbsp capers
- 2 tbsp olive oil
- 2 tbsp fresh parsley, chopped
- 1/2 tsp pepper

Greek vinaigrette
- 1/4 cup olive oil
- 2 tbsp red wine vinegar
- 1 tbsp lemon juice
- 1/2 tsp garlic powder
- 1 tsp dried oregano
- 1/2 tsp kosher salt
- 1/2 tsp ground black pepper

INSTRUCTIONS:
1. Combine all the ingredients for the Greek vinaigrette and shake well.
2. Grill sausages according to package directions. Cut in half, then quarters and set aside.

3. In a bowl, add pepper, olive oil, zucchini, squash, and tomatoes. Grill or cook for 5 minutes.
4. Add sausages, vinaigrette, capers, olives, and parsley. Then toss with the vegetables.
5. Serve and enjoy!

TACO MEAL PREP BOWLS

Prep Time: 5 minutes
Cook Time: 10 minutes
Total Time: 15 minutes
Serves: 8

***INGREDIENTS*:**
- 2 c brown rice (cooked)
- 2 tablespoon olive oil
- 2 pounds ground beef
- 1 tablespoon Chili Powder
- 1/4 teaspoon Garlic Powder
- 1/4 teaspoon Onion Powder
- 1/4 teaspoon Red Pepper Flakes (crushed)
- 1/4 teaspoon Dried Oregano
- 1/2 teaspoon Paprika
- 1 1/2 teaspoon Cumin
- 1 teaspoon Salt
- 1 teaspoon Black Pepper
- 1/2 cup salsa verde

- 2 cups black beans (drained, rinsed)
- 2 cups whole kernel corn, drained
- 4 Roma tomatoes (diced, sliced into chunks)
- Fresh cilantro (for garnish)
- Lime wedges (for garnish)

INSTRUCTIONS:

1. In a skillet, add olive oil and place over medium-high heat.
2. Add ground beef break it up to crumble.
3. Add all the seasonings and stir well.
4. Add the salsa verde and combine.
5. Remove from heat and remove excess grease.
6. Divide rice into 8 containers.
7. Divide tomatoes, corn, black beans and beef mixture into the 8 containers.
8. Sprinkle cilantro and lime to squeeze.
9. Stays 5 days in the fridge.

Loaded Breakfast Stuffed Peppers

Prep Time: 10 minutes
Cook Time: 25 minutes
Total Time: **35 minutes**
Serves: 8

INGREDIENTS

- 4 L bell peppers (seeded, cut widthwise)
- 9 L eggs (beaten)
- 1/2 c breakfast potatoes (fully cooked)
- 1/2 c quinoa (cooked)
- 1/2 c black beans
- 1/2 c spinach leaves (chopped)
- 1/3 c shredded cheese plus more for toppings
- 1 tsp salt
- 1/4 tsp black pepper

INSTRUCTIONS:

1. Preheat the oven to 400°F. Put the peppers on a baking sheet and bake for about 5 minutes.
2. In a bowl with beaten eggs, add the remaining ingredients and mix well to combine.
3. Remove peppers from oven and spoon egg mixture into peppers.
4. Sprinkle with cheese and bake for 30 minutes.
5. Serve immediately.

Greek Quinoa Breakfast Bowl

Prep Time: 10 minutes
Cook Time: 20 minutes
Total Time: 30 minutes
Serves: 5

INGREDIENTS:
12 eggs
¼ c plain greek yogurt
1 tsp onion powder
1 tsp granulated garlic
½ tsp salt
½ tsp pepper
1 tsp olive oil
1 (5 oz) bag baby spinach
1 pint cherry tomatoes (halved)
1 c feta cheese
2 c cooked quinoa

INSTRUCTIONS:

1. In a bowl, add eggs, salt and pepper, granulated garlic, onion powder, greek yogurt, and granulated garlic. Whisk and set aside.
2. In a skillet, add olive oil over medium heat and add spinach. Cook for 3 minutes.

3. Add egg mixture and cook for 7 minutes. Scramble the eggs to set.
4. Add quinoa and feta then cook to heat through.
5. Serve immediately.

Spinach, Feta and Egg Breakfast Quesadillas

Prep Time: 10 minutes
Cook Time: 15 minutes
Total Time: 25 minutes
Serves: 4

INGREDIENTS:

spray oil
2 tsp olive oil
1/2 red onion
1 red bell pepper
8 eggs
1/4 c milk
1/4 teaspoon salt
1/4 teaspoon pepper
4 handfuls of spinach leaves
1/2 c feta
1 1/2 c mozzarella cheese
5 tortillas

INSTRUCTIONS:

1. In a non-stick pan, add oil and place over medium heat.
2. Add red onion and bell pepper, then cook for 4 minutes.
3. In a bowl. Whisk the milk, eggs, and salt and pepper.
4. Pour egg mixture into the pan together with pepper and onion. Stir until eggs are just cooked through.
5. Add feta and spinach, and cook until wilted.
6. Remove from the heat.
7. In a separate pan, spray oil and place over medium heat.
8. Add tortilla. Spread a half cup of egg mixture into half of the tortilla. Top with ⅓ cup cheese and fold. Cook for 2 minutes.
9. Flip and cook for another minute.

Teriyaki Chicken and Broccoli

Prep Time: 5 minutes
Cook Time: 15 minutes
Total Time: 20 minutes
Serves: 4

INGREDIENTS:
- 1 lb chicken breasts (boneless, skinless, cut into bite-sized pieces)
- salt and pepper
- 1 tbsp oil

- 2 c broccoli florets
- 1 bell pepper (stripped)
- sesame seeds (for garnish)
- 2 cups brown rice (cooked)

For the teriyaki sauce:
- 1/4 c light soy sauce
- 2 tbsp honey
- 2 tbsp rice wine vinegar
- 1 tbsp cornstarch
- 1 clove minced garlic
- 1/2 tsp sesame oil
- 1/4 tsp ground ginger

INSTRUCTIONS:

1. Place a pan over medium-high heat and add chicken seasoned with salt and pepper, Cook for 3 minutes.
2. To make teriyaki sauce, whisk all the ingredients in a bowl.
3. Pour teriyaki sauce over chicken and cook for 4 minutes. Transfer chicken to a bowl.
4. Add bell pepper and broccoli to the pan and stir-fry for 2 minutes.
5. Divide broccoli and chicken into 4 containers. Add a half cup of rice into each meal prep container.
6. Garnish with sesame seed on top.
7. Can stay 4 days in the fridge.

Quinoa Egg Breakfast Muffin Recipe

Prep Time: 10 minutes
Cook Time: 30 minutes
Total Time: 40 minutes
Serves: 4

INGREDIENTS:

6 eggs
1/4 teaspoon pepper
1/4 teaspoon salt
1 c cooked quinoa
3/4 c cheese (shredded)
1 c mushrooms sliced
1/2 onion
1/2 c sundried tomatoes (drained, chopped)
¼ shredded cheese (toppings)

INSTRUCTIONS:

1. Preheat the oven to 350°F.
2. In a bowl, add eggs, and salt and pepper then whisk.
3. Add the remaining ingredients (except cheese for toppings) and stir.
4. Spoon mixture into muffin pan with muffin liners.
5. Sprinkle shredded cheese on top.
6. Bake for 20 minutes.

Peanut butter & jam breakfast cookies

Prep Time: 10 minutes
Cook Time: 15 minutes
Total Time: 25 minutes
Serves: 5

INGREDIENTS:
2 tbsp coconut oil (melted)
2/3 c natural peanut butter
2 L eggs
1/2 tsp vanilla
1/4 c honey
1/2 c rolled oats
1/2 c all-purpose flour
1/2 tsp baking powder
1/4 c ground flax
6 tbsp jam of choice

INSTRUCTIONS:

1. Heat the oven to 350°F.
2. Line a baking sheet with parchment papers.
3. In a bowl, add the melted coconut oil, honey, vanilla, eggs and peanut butter. Stir until smooth.
4. Add ground flax, baking powder, flour and rolled oats. Mix well to combine.

5. Scoop ¼ cup of mixture and shape to a round cookie. Place on the baking sheet and make a hole in the middle.
6. Spoon a tablespoon of jam into the hole of each round cookie.
7. Bake for 13 minutes.
8. Cool before storing.

Healthy Freezer Breakfast Sandwiches

Prep Time: 10 minutes
Cook Time: 20 minutes
Total Time: 30 minutes
Serves: 4

INGREDIENTS:

6 eggs
1/4 c milk
1/8 tsp salt
1/2 c feta crumbled
1 1/2 c spinach (chopped)
1 1/2 c broccoli (finely chopped)
4 slices Havarti
4 whole wheat English muffins

INSTRUCTIONS:

1. Heat the oven to 375°F.
2. Spray baking dish with spray oil.
3. In a bowl, add the milk and the eggs then beat together. Fold in the feta, salt, broccoli, and spinach.
4. Pour the egg mixture into the prepared baking dish.
5. Bake for 20 minutes.
6. Cool completely and then cut into 4 circles.
7. Add one egg and cheese between muffin.
8. Wrap in a ziplock can stay in the fridge for 4 days.

Maple Apple Steel Cut Oats

Prep Time: 5 minutes
Cook Time: 25 minutes
Total Time: 30 minutes
Serves: 5

INGREDIENTS:
1 c steel cut oats
1 c unsweetened applesauce
3 c water
1 L apple (cut into small pieces)
1 tsp ground cinnamon
1/2 tsp ground cardamom
2 tsp maple extract
After cooking
2 tbsp maple syrup
1/3 c chopped pecans

INSTRUCTIONS:

1. In a pot, add all the ingredients and combine by stirring. Cook over medium heat.
2. Bring to a boil and turn the heat to low. Cover and simmer for 20 minutes.
3. Garnish with chopped pecans and drizzle maple syrup.

Healthy Chicken and Veggies

Prep Time: 10 minutes
Cook Time: 20 minutes
Total Time: 30 minutes
Serves: 4

INGREDIENTS:
- 2 M chicken breasts (boneless, skinless, cut into half-inch pieces)
- 1 c fresh broccoli florets
- 1 S red onion (chopped)
- 1 c grape
- 1 M zucchini (chopped)
- 2 cloves minced garlic
- 1 tbsp Italian seasoning
- 1 tsp salt
- 1/2 tsp black pepper
- 1/2 tsp red pepper flakes

- 1/2 tsp paprika
- 2 tbsp olive oil
- 2 c cooked rice of choice

INSTRUCTIONS:

1. Preheat the oven to 450°F. Line a baking sheet using aluminum foil.
2. Place veggies and chicken into the baking sheet.
3. Sprinkle all the garlic and spices evenly.
4. Drizzle with olive oil.
5. Bake for 20 minutes.
6. Place a half cup of rice to each 4 meal prep containers.
7. Divide veggies and chicken over rice.
8. Cover and stays up in the fridge for 5 days.

BANANA ZUCCHINI OATMEAL CUPS

Prep Time: 15 minutes
Cook Time: 25 minutes
Total Time: 40 minutes
Serves: 4

INGREDIENTS:

1 tablespoon ground flaxseed plus 3 tablespoon water
¼ cup almond butter
¼ cup maple syrup

3 M over-ripe bananas (mashed)
2 S zucchinis (grated, do not squeeze)
½ cup almond milk
1 teaspoon vanilla extract
3 cups old-fashioned oats
1 tablespoon baking powder
1 teaspoon cinnamon
¼ teaspoon salt

INSTRUCTIONS:
1. Preheat the oven to 375°F.
2. In the muffin tin line with muffin liners.
3. In a bowl, add water and flax. Stir and set aside
4. In a bowl, add bananas, flax mixture, maple syrup, almond butter, vanilla extract, almond milk, and zucchini. Stir well to combine.
5. Add salt, cinnamon, baking powder and oats. Stir well to combined.
6. Spoon mixture into prepared muffin tin.
7. Bake for 25 minutes.
8. Store in an air-tight container.

Strawberry Banana Baked Oatmeal

Prep Time: 10 minutes
Cook Time: 35 minutes
Total Time: 45 minutes
Serves: 8

INGREDIENTS:
3 M ripe banana (mashed)
2 eggs
3 c milk
¼ c pure maple syrup
2 tsp vanilla extract
1 tsp cinnamon
1 tsp baking powder
½ tsp salt
4 c old-fashioned oats
1 ½ c strawberries (chopped plus more for serving

INSTRUCTIONS:

1. Preheat the oven to 350°F. Grease a baking dish.
2. In a bowl, add baking powder, salt, cinnamon, vanilla, maple syrup, milk, eggs and mashed bananas. Whisk together.
3. Stir in the strawberries and oats.
4. Pour the mixture into the baking dish.
5. Bake for 35 minutes.
6. Let cool for 5 minutes.
7. Serve with strawberries on top.

Part 2

Introduction

There should be something for almost anyone within these pages, whether you are new to meal prepping or a seasoned professional. You can check out the book based on the main ingredient, or browse through and see if any specific recipes catch your eye. All of the dishes are fresh, healthy and easy, and sure to help you on your way to becoming the best meal prepper you can be.

Just a small note: Most of the recipes contain nutritional information, but unfortunately it is not available for all of them. As much as it would be ideal to include them, it is not totally possible for all, but where it is possible, we have made sure to do so for you.

There are plenty of books on this subject on the market, thanks again for choosing this one! Every effort was made to ensure it is full of as many useful recipes and yummy dishes as possible, so please enjoy!

Chapter 1: Salad Recipes

When you are trying to eat healthy, salads are an obvious choice in helping you on your way to your goals. Many people think that salads are either too light to be a meal or not filling enough on their own to last you until the next meal. However, if you are making salads with additional proteins and toppings added in, then they are a great way to stay feeling full while also avoiding consuming any unnecessary or unwanted extra calories and fats. In this chapter, several different types of salads will be detailed, as well as less traditional versions of the classic, healthy dish.

Flavorful Chef's Salad

For this dish, you can expect to produce 4 servings, with an estimated time of around 25 minutes for any preparation, along with around 25 minutes of cooking or baking the ingredients.

What is in it:
- Salt and pepper (coarse, ground)
- Monterey Jack cheese (4 oz. Sliced into strips)
- Carrots (4, shredded)
- Radishes (6, diced)
- Alfalfa sprouts (1 cup)
- Avocado (1, cut)
- Roasted turkey breast (1 lbs., cut)

- Lettuce (1 head)
- Cider vinegar (2 tbsp.)
- Honey (1 tbsp.)
- Low-fat buttermilk (.3 cup)
- Low-fat sour cream (.3 cup)

How it is done:
- Using a bowl or mixing dish, place your buttermilk, honey, sour cream, and vinegar together, then add your salt and pepper to your own personal taste. Once all ingredients are mixed, feel free to place this off to the side.
- Chop your lettuce up then split it into four different servings. Spread the rest of your toppings—turkey, avocado, radishes, sprouts, cheese, and carrots—on top.
- Spread your dressing mix on top of the lettuce mix.

Buttery Lettuce with Egg and Potato

For this dish, you can expect to produce 4 servings, with an estimated time of around 40 minutes for any preparation, along with around 55 minutes of cooking or baking the ingredients.

What is in it:
- Fresh chives (.25 cup)
- Eggs (4, fried)

- Lemon juice (2 tbsp.)
- Butter lettuce (1-2 heads, chopped)
- Sugar (.25 tsp.)
- Unsalted butter (1 stick)
- Asparagus (16 oz., sliced)
- Sugar snap peas (.5 lbs., cut in half)
- Salt and pepper (added to your taste)
- Baby potatoes (16 oz.)

How it is done:
- Place your potatoes into a pot or large baking dish and add enough water to lightly submerge the potatoes. Heat the water until it begins to boil, then add in some salt. Continue cooking the potatoes in this water until they are tender and easily cut into, then scoop them out of the pot, leaving the water to keep boiling.
- Place your snap peas and asparagus into the same pot as the potatoes and allow them to continue boiling until the reach a tender state, soft or around 2 minutes. Remove them from the stove then strain out the water.
- Cut your potatoes into .25 inch slices.
- Place a pan on your stove, then add in your butter and let it melt in the heat. Once it is melted, take it off of the stove and mix in your lemon juice and sugar, adding salt and pepper as well.
- Split you lettuce and vegetables into 4 different portions, then add you dressing mixture and eggs. Season as you see fit.

Chicken Salad with Almonds and Green Beans

For this dish, you can expect to produce 4 servings, with an estimated time of around 30 minutes for any preparation, along with around 30 minutes of cooking or baking the ingredients.

What is in it:
- Almonds (.25 cup, chopped)
- Baby arugula (5 oz.)
- Radicchio (1 head, sliced)
- Green beans (8 oz.)
- Red-wine vinegar (2 tbsp.)
- Salt and pepper (to your own taste)
- Chicken breast, boneless skinless (16 oz.)
- Olive oil (3 tbsp.)
- Apricot jam (1 tbsp.)
- Dijon mustard (1 tbsp.)

How it is made:
- Using a pan, pour 1 tablespoon of your olive oil in and heat on high. Place your chicken breast in the pan, salting and peppering before you cook. Allow the chicken to cook on either side for around 2-3 minutes, then cut once cooled.
- Boil water for your green beans, adding a little bit of salt to the water before the beans go in. Once the water is boiling, add in your green beans and cook

them for 5-6 minutes while covered. Strain the beans and run them under some colder water to cool.
- Using a smaller bowl, mix your jam, vinegar, mustard, and the rest of your olive oil with some salt and pepper.
- Add your greens to another bowl and mix together with 2/3 o your dressing. Separate out your greens, then add the rest of your toppings and drizzle on what is left of the dressing.

Chicken, Pistachio, and Feta Salad

For this dish, you can expect to produce 4 servings, with an estimated time of around 30 minutes for any preparation, along with around 30 minutes of cooking or baking the ingredients.

What is in it:
- Oranges (2, peeled and separated)
- Feta cheese (4 oz.)
- Scallions (1 bunch, cut)
- Romaine lettuce (1 head, sliced)
- Parsley (.5 cup)
- Chicken cutlet, boneless skinless (16 oz.)
- Ground Coriander (1 tsp.)
- Salt and pepper (to your own taste)
- White-wine vinegar).25 cup)
- Olive oil (.25 cup)
- Pistachios (.5 cup, unsalted)

How it is done:
- Using a medium-sized pan, place your pistachios in and allow to roast over a medium level of heat. Stir them often for around 7-8 minutes. Remove them from the burner, then allow them to cool.
- Mix together your oil and vinegar in another bowl, adding in your salt and pepper.
- Pour two tablespoons of oil into another pan. Season your chicken with the coriander and salt and pepper, then add to the skillet, cooking on both sides for around 3-4 minutes. Once the chicken is cooked and cooled, cut it into thin slices.
- Place your pistachios, scallions, lettuce, and parsley into a bowl, adding in your homemade dressing, mixing until they are combined. Finish the dish off by topping with chicken, feta and orange slices.

Turkey Taco Salad

For this dish, you can expect to produce 6 servings, with an estimated time of around 20 minutes for any preparation, along with around 30 minutes of cooking or baking the ingredients.

What is in it:
- Your choice of shredded cheese (1 cup)
- Cherry tomatoes (1 cup, cut)
- Tortilla chips (1.5 cups, crushed)

- Lettuce (2 heads)
- Salt and pepper (to your own taste)
- Your choice of salsa (1.5 cups)
- Red Bell Pepper (1, chopped)
- Zucchini (1, chopped)
- Ground turkey (16 oz.)
- Onion (1, chopped)
- Olive oil (4 tbsp.)

How it is done:
- Allow two tablespoons of your olive oil to heat over the stove, then sprinkle in the chopped onion and cook, making sure to stir often, for around 6-7 minutes total. Once the onions are done, also place your turkey into the same skillet, again making sure to stir often, for another 6-7 minutes.
- Once your turkey is done, mix in your zucchini, half your salsa, and the bell pepper, allowing the mixture to continue cooking for another 4-6 minutes.
- In another bowl, mix your lettuce, tomatoes, tortilla chip chunks and the rest of your salsa together with 1-2 tablespoons of olive oil. Once the mixture is done, place your turkey and veggies on top and sprinkle cheese on to finish.

Spinach Salad with Salmon

For this dish, you can expect to produce 4 servings, with an estimated time of around 10 minutes for any preparation, along with around 15 minutes of cooking or baking the ingredients.

What is in it:
- Balsamic Vinaigrette (.25 cup)
- Pecans (.25 cup)
- Goat cheese (.75 cup, crumbled)
- Grape tomatoes(1 pint, cut)
- Baby spinach (10 oz.)
- Salt and pepper (to your own taste)
- Salmon fillet (24 oz., skinless)

How it is done:
- Allow your broiler to heat up, setting your rack somewhere around 4 inches away from the heat source. Line or fill a baking pan with foil in order to catch any juice, then put your salmon fillets on the pan, using salt and pepper as you see fit.
- Allow the salmon to broil for around 8-9 minutes. Once the salmon has had time to cool, cut it into smaller pieces.
- Split the rest of your solid ingredients up into portions. Place the salmon on top and spread your vinaigrette on to finish.

Steak and Arugula Salad

For this dish, you can expect to produce 4 servings, with an estimated time of around 30 minutes for any preparation, along with around 30 minutes of cooking or baking the ingredients.

What is in it:
- Goat cheese (2 oz,)
- Arugula (3 bunches)
- Salsa (1 cup)
- Flank steak (16 oz.)
- Balsamic vinegar (2 tsp.)
- Olive oil (2 tsp.)
- Salt and pepper (to your own taste)
- Ground cumin (.5 tsp.)
- Chili powder (2 tsp.)
- Dried oregano (.5 tsp.)

How it is made:
- Mix together your cumin, chili powder, .5 teaspoons of salt and oregano, then coat your steak with the seasoning mixture.
- Cook your steak in a pan with heated oil, allowing it to cook on each side for around 5-7 minutes or once it reaches the rarity level that you desire. Allow your steak to cool for a little bit then cut it into slices.
- Mix your salsa and vinegar together, adding in some salt and pepper as you see fit. Place Your arugula into this mixture and coat.
- Spilt all of your ingredients up into four portions,

then finish it off with some goat cheese as a topping.

Rice and Black Bean Salad with Chicken

For this dish, you can expect to produce 4 servings, with an estimated time of around 25 minutes for any preparation, along with around 60 minutes of cooking or baking the ingredients.

What is in it:
- Scallions (4, chopped)
- Olive oil (3 tbsp.)
- Salt and pepper (to your own taste)
- Jalapeno chili (1, chopped)
- White-wine vinegar (.25 cup)
- Ground cumin (.5 tsp.)
- Plum tomatoes (6, sliced)
- Rice (1 cup, brown or white)
- Black Beans (1 can, washed)
- Chicken (2.5 lbs, cooked and cut)

How it is done:
- Allow your rice to cook based off of the directions on the package, then place the rice into your fridge to let it cool off.
- Once the rice has cooled completely, add it to a large bowl with your chicken, scallions, beans, tomatoes,

vinegar, oil, jalapeno, and cumin. Mix the ingredients together and sprinkle with salt and pepper.

Lite Cobb Salad

For this dish, you can expect to produce 4 servings, with an estimated time of around 20 minutes for any preparation, along with around 20 minutes of cooking or baking the ingredients.

What is in it:
- Avocado (1, cut)
- Eggs (4, hard-boiled and cut)
- Plum tomatoes (4, cut)
- Deli turkey (6 oz., cut)
- Lettuce (2 heads, sliced)
- Salt
- Blue cheese (.5 cup)
- Red-wine vinegar (1 tbsp.)
- Mayonnaise (.25 cup, light)
- Low-fat buttermilk (1 cup)
- Turkey bacon (3 slices)

How it is done:
- Cook up your turkey bacon for around 6-7 minutes in a pan without any oil, then place on a paper towel to soak up some of the grease, splitting it into small

pieces.
- Mix the buttermilk, vinegar, and mayo together, then fold in the blue cheese bits. Salt as you see fit.
- Place the lettuce as your base, then add the rest of your toppings and dressing.

Shrimp and Cucumber Salad

For this dish, you can expect to produce 4 servings, with an estimated time of around 30 minutes for any preparation, along with around 30 minutes of cooking or baking the ingredients.

What is in it:
- Olive oil (4 tsp.)
- Dried oregano (.25 tsp.)
- Ground coriander (.5 tsp.)
- Ground cumin (1 tsp.)
- Shrimp (16 oz, medium size, cleaned)
- Salt and pepper (to your own taste)
- Red-wine vinegar (2 tbsp.)
- Orange juice (.25 cup)
- Hearts of palm (1 can, strained and sliced)
- Jalapeno pepper (1, diced)
- Red onion (.5, chopped)
- Cucumber (.5, peeled and sliced)

How it is done:
- Add your cucumber, jalapeno, orange juice, onion, hearts of palm, and vinegar to a bowl, then add salt

and pepper to your own liking.
- Sprinkle your cumin, coriander, and oregano over the shrimp, as well as some salt and pepper.
- Place the shrimp in a pan with heated oil and cook on each side of the shrimp for around 3-4 minutes.
- Place your shrimp over top of the cucumber mixture and serve.

Ham, Egg, and Spinach Salad

For this dish, you can expect to produce 4 servings, with an estimated time of around 25 minutes for any preparation, along with around 25 minutes of cooking or baking the ingredients.

What is in it:
- Eggs (6 hard-boiled, cut)
- Spinach (16 oz., chopped)
- Radishes (6, chopped)
- Ham (8 oz, chopped)
- Grainy mustard (2 tsp.)
- Salt and pepper (to your own taste)
- White-wine vinegar (2 tbsp.)
- Onion (1, chopped)
- Olive oil (6 tbsp.)

How it is made:

- Cook your onion up in heated oil. Once it has cooked for 5-6 minute, take it off of the stove and mix in your vinegar, .75 teaspoons of salt, mustard and .25 teaspoons of pepper.
- With your ham, egg, and spinach acting as a base, toss in your radishes then pour in the onion mixture.

White-bean Shrimp Salad

For this dish, you can expect to produce 4 servings, with an estimated time of around 20 minutes for any preparation, along with around 20 minutes of cooking or baking the ingredients.

What is in it:
- Lettuce or your choice of leafy greens (8 oz.)
- Grainy mustard (1 tsp.)
- Cannellini beans (2 cans, washed)
- White-wine vinegar (1.5 tbsp.)
- Olive oil (3 tbsp.)
- Dried marjoram (.5 tsp.)
- Salt and pepper (to your own taste)
- Bacon (4 oz.)
- Shrimp (16 oz., peeled and cleaned)

How it is made:
- Slice your bacon into smaller pieces, then allow it to cook, adding in your shrimp once the bacon has turned golden. Cook for another 5 minutes then take

off of the burner and place into a bowl.
- In another bowl mix your oil, mustard, marjoram, and vinegar together.
- Add the beans and lettuce or leafy greens to the shrimp and bacon mix, then finish it off with the vinaigrette.

Mediterranean Salad

For this dish, you can expect to produce 4 servings, with an estimated time of around 35 minutes for any preparation, along with around 35 minutes of cooking or baking the ingredients.

What is in it:
- Feta cheese (4 oz.)
- Cannellini beans (1 can, washed)
- Olive oil (2 tbsp.)
- Artichoke hearts (1 can, sliced)
- Dijon mustard (1 tbsp.)
- Romaine lettuce (1 head, cut)
- Red-wine vinegar (2 tbsp)
- Sun-dried tomatoes (.25 cup, sliced)
- Salt and pepper (to your own taste)
- Penne pasta (1 cup)

How it is made:
- Allow your pasta to cook according to the directions

on the package, but add in your sun-dried tomatoes one minute or so before the pasta reaches al dente, then cook for another minute and strain. Allow the pasta to sit under cold water for a few seconds, then strain again.
- For the dressing, mix together the mustard, vinegar, 1 tablespoon of water and oil, then add salt and pepper to your own liking.
- Mix all of your ingredients together and serve.

Chicken and Mango Salad

For this dish, you can expect to produce 4 servings, with an estimated time of around 25 minutes for any preparation, along with around 25 minutes of cooking or baking the ingredients.

What is in it:
- Mango (1, peeled and chopped)
- Salt and pepper (to your own taste)
- Baby spinach (10 oz.)
- Cayenne pepper (.25 tsp.)
- Rotisserie chicken (4 cups, shredded)
- Ground turmeric (1 tsp.)
- Cilantro (.5 cup, chopped)
- Dijon mustard (1 tbsp.)
- Lime juice (2 tbsp.)
- Mango chutney (2 tbsp.)

- Sweetened shredded coconut (.5 cup)
- Low-fat yogurt (.75 cup)

How it is made:
- Allow your oven to heat up to 350F. Sprinkle the coconut onto a baking pan and put it into the oven for 6-8 minutes, then allow it to sit and cool.
- Place all of your other ingredients together and mix, except for the chicken and mango. Once the mixture is combined, add in your chicken and mango, then top with the coconut over and serve over some spinach.

Asian Rotisserie Chicken Salad

For this dish, you can expect to produce 4 servings, with an estimated time of around 30 minutes for any preparation, along with around 30 minutes of cooking or baking the ingredients.

What is in it:
- Romaine lettuce (1 head, cut)
- Cashews (.5 cup)
- Red bell pepper (1, chopped)
- Rotisserie chicken (4 cups, shredded)
- Scallions (2, chopped)

- Red cabbage (.25, chopped)
- Vegetable oil (.25 cup)
- Salt and pepper (to your own taste)
- Cilantro (2 cups)
- Lime juice (.25 cup)

How it is done:
- Using a blender or food processor, add the lime juice, cilantro, and oil together and blend, Add salt and pepper to your own liking.
- Mix together your bell pepper, chicken, scallions, and cabbage, then add salt and pepper to your own liking.
- Mix your lettuce together with .5 cups of your dressing mixture, then split your ingredients up and cover with the rest of the dressing. Add the cashews to the top to finish.

Romaine, Avocado, and Tuna Salad

For this dish, you can expect to produce 4 servings, with an estimated time of around 15 minutes for any preparation, along with around 15 minutes of cooking or baking the ingredients.

What is in it:
- Avocado (1, chopped)

- Romaine lettuce (1 head, cut)
- Salt and pepper (to your own taste)
- Radishes (1 bunch, cut)
- Tuna (2 cans)
- Dijon mustard (1 tbsp.)
- Olive oil (.3 cups)
- White-wine vinegar (3 tbsp.)

What is in it:
- Mix the vinegar, olive oil and mustard together with your choice of salt and pepper added.
- In another bowl, add your tuna, avocado, radishes, and lettuce together.
- Pour dressing over the mixture and mix together. Top off with pepper then serve.

Citrus-Infused Steak Salad

For this dish, you can expect to produce 4 servings, with an estimated time of around 20 minutes for any preparation, along with around 20 minutes of cooking or baking the ingredients.

What is in it:
- Onion (1, diced)
- Romaine lettuce (1 head, sliced)
- Carrots (4, sliced thinly)

- Ginger (1 tsp., grated)
- Vegetable oil (2 tbsp.)
- Honey (2 tbsp.)
- Salt and pepper (to your own taste)
- Oranges (2, peeled and split)
- Strip steak (4, 20 oz. total)

How it is done:
- Add salt and pepper to your steak and then place in a pan with oil. Allow the steak to cook for around 8-10 minutes, making sure to flip it over once. Once the steak has had time to cool, slice it into thin pieces.
- Add some zest from the orange peels to a bowl, then mix in with some oil, ginger, and honey. Once the mixture is mixed, place the lettuce, carrots, onion and orange pieces into the mixture, then top with steak.

Soba Noodle Salad with Chicken

For this dish, you can expect to produce 4 servings, with an estimated time of around 10 minutes for any preparation, along with around 15 minutes of cooking or baking the ingredients.

What is in it:
- Red cabbage (2.25 cups, diced)
- Ginger (1 tsp., grated)

- Scallions (6, chopped)
- Sugar (1 tsp.)
- Chicken (.12 oz., cooked and shredded)
- Rice vinegar (2 tbsp.)
- Garlic (1 clove, minced)
- Vegetable oil (1 tbsp.)
- Gluten-free soba (12 oz.)
- Gluten-free soy sauce (.25 cup)

How it is done:
- Place the soba into a pot and cook by following the direction on the soba package.
- Mix together the soy sauce, sugar, vinegar, garlic, oil, and garlic until it has all combined evenly.
- Once the noodles have finished cooking, strain them, run them under cold water, then strain them again.
- Mix your noodles with your soy sauce mixture, then finish by adding in the chicken, cabbage, and scallions.

Tortilla, Bean, and Corn Salad

For this dish, you can expect to produce 4 servings, with an estimated time of around 25 minutes for any preparation, along with around 25 minutes of cooking or baking the ingredients.

What is in it:

- Pepper jack cheese (.75 cup, grated)
- Salt and pepper (to your own taste)
- Tortilla chips (3 cups, crushed)
- Romaine hearts (1 bag, chopped)
- Avocado (1, sliced)
- Salsa (.25 cup)
- Plum tomatoes (3, cut)
- Scallions (1 bunch, chopped)
- Pinto beans (1 can, washed)
- Frozen corn (1 package, around 2 cups)

How it is done:
- Add the salsa, beans, and corn to a bowl, then put in the microwave for around 1 minute. Once the mix is warm throughout, add the tomatoes, scallions, and avocado with some salt and pepper.
- In another bowl, put your lettuce and chips together and mix. Scoop your bean mixture onto the lettuce as a topping, then sprinkle on cheese to finish.

Tuna, Celery, and Cucumber Salad

For this dish, you can expect to produce 4 servings, with an estimated time of around 10 minutes for any preparation, along with around 10 minutes of cooking or baking the ingredients.

What is in it:
- Salt and pepper (to your own taste)
- Cucumbers (2, sliced)
- Tuna (2 cans, drained)
- Extra-virgin olive oil (2 tbsp.)
- Celery (3 stalks, sliced)
- Sugar (1 tbsp)
- Poppy seeds (2 tsp.)
- Rice vinegar (3 tbsp.)

How it is made:
- Grab a bowl and mix your sugar, poppy seeds, vinegar, and oil together, then add in the tuna, cucumbers, and celery as well, making sure to season with whatever amount of salt and pepper you would like. Mix the ingredients together well, then garnish with celery leaves to finish.

Chapter 2: Chicken Recipes

Chicken is one of the most common and versatile main ingredient in many different healthy dishes. By combining different seasonings and sauces, you can turn chicken into virtually any sort of dish you can imagine. In this chapter, we will cover chicken recipes that feature a wide variety of flavors and mixtures but are all relatively healthy and easy to make, too.

Grilled Chicken and Roasted Kale

For this dish, you can expect to produce 4 servings, with an estimated time of around 10 minutes for any preparation, along with around 30 minutes of cooking or baking the ingredients.

Each serving includes:

14 g Fat

28 g Carbohydrates

50 g Protein

What is in it:

- Lemon juice (1 tbsp.)
- Cherry tomatoes (.5 cup, sliced)
- Chicken breast, skinless boneless (2, halved)
- Parmesan cheese (.3 cup)
- Salt and pepper (to your own taste)
- Kale (1 bunch, only leaves)
- Extra-virgin olive oil (2 tbsp.)
- Garlic (3 cloves, minced)
- Red-skinned potatoes (8 oz., small, sliced)

How it is done:

- Be sure to set your oven to 425F before starting.
- Mix your potatoes with .5 tablespoons of oil, then place in a baking pan and cook in the oven for five minutes.
- Mix the kale with the same amount of olive oil, .25 teaspoons of salt, garlic, and pepper. Put the kale with the potatoes and allow them both to cook for another 15-20 minutes.
- Either grill your chicken or cook over the stove for 4-5 minutes on each side, coating with .5 tablespoons of olive oil, salt, and pepper.
- Add the kale, potatoes, olive oil left, leafy greens, lemon juice, tomatoes, salt, and pepper and parmesan together, then place chicken on top.

Homemade Chicken Fingers

For this dish, you can expect to produce 4 servings, with an estimated time of around 20 minutes for any preparation, along with around 20 minutes of cooking or baking the ingredients.

Each serving includes:

6 g Fat

38 g Protein

What is in it:

- Chicken tenders or boneless skinless chicken breast (2 lbs.)
- Egg whites (2)
- Salt
- Sweet paprika (.5 tsp.)
- Parsley (1 tbsp., chopped)
- Parmesan (.3 cup, grated)
- Cornflake cereal (2 cups)
- Whole wheat melba toast (2 oz.)

How it is done:

- Take the cornflakes, melba toast, parsley, paprika, parmesan, and .5 teaspoons of salt in a bag and

crush. Place the crushed mixture into a bowl or dish, then in another bowl mix together the egg whites and 2 tablespoons of water.
- Take the chicken tenders or sliced chicken breasts and coat them in the egg white mix, then dip into the cornflake mix. Once they are all coated, bake them at 425F for 18-20 minutes.
- Remove from the oven and serve, or freeze for later use.

Marinated Chicken Breasts

For this dish, you can expect to produce 4 servings, with an estimated time of around 5 minutes for any preparation, along with around 8 hours of cooking or baking the ingredients.

Each serving includes:

16 g Fat

3 g Carbohydrates

40 g Protein

What is in it:

- Chicken breast, boneless skinless (4)
- Extra-virgin olive oil (.25 up)

- Dijon mustard (1-2 tbsp.)
- Salt and pepper (to your own taste)
- Garlic powder (1-2 tsp.)
- Vinegar (1-2 tbsp.)
- Oregano and rosemary (2-3 tsp.)

How it is done:

- In a bag, combine the herbs, vinegar, mustard, and oil and shake. Place the chicken breasts into the bag, shake, then freeze. Allow the chicken to freeze for at least a few days, but also up to 2 weeks.
- Take the chicken out of the freezer once time has passed and allow it to thaw out using your choice of a method.
- Preheat your grill for around ten minutes, then place the chicken on and cook for around 4 minutes on each side, or for around 15 minutes in the oven at 375F.
- Serve with your choice of sides or veggies.

Apple-Honey Drumsticks

For this dish, you can expect to produce 6 servings, with an estimated time of around 20 minutes for any preparation, along with around 40 minutes of cooking or baking the ingredients.

Each serving includes:

13 g Fat

21 g Protein

65 g Carbohydrates

What is in it:

- Drumsticks (12)
- Butter (1 tbsp., unsalted)
- Sesame seeds (2 tsps.)
- Red pepper flakes (.25 tsp.)
- Lemon zest (1 lemon's worth)
- Honey (2 tsp.)
- Soy sauce (.25 cup)
- Apple juice (2 cups)
- Salt and pepper (to taste)
- Apple cider vinegar (.5 cup)

How it is done:

- Before you begin, make sure to set your oven to 450F.
- Place a wire rack onto a baking pan, then place the chicken on top of it and use salt and pepper to season.
- Place your drumsticks into the oven for 30 minutes, then turn to the other side and let cook for another 30 minutes.

- For the sauce, put the ingredients in a pot and let simmer on high: apple juice, honey, vinegar, lemon zest, soy sauce, red pepper flakes, and a sprinkle of salt. Let it stay on the stove until it develops a syrupy texture, likely around 20-25 minutes. Add the sesame seeds and allow it to cool a little.
- Place your chicken into a bowl large enough to hold the chicken and the sauce, then mix in the sauce along with some butter, allowing it to coat the chicken.

Honey-Mustard Chicken with Apples

For this dish, you can expect to produce 4 servings, with an estimated time of around 10 minutes for any preparation, along with around 30 minutes of cooking or baking the ingredients.

Each serving includes:

- 28 g Fat

- 33 g Protein

- 18 g Carbohydrates

What is in it:
- Parsley (1-2 tbsp.)

- Unsalted butter (1.5 tsp.)
- Chicken broth (1 cup)
- All-purpose flour (1 tbsp.)
- Honey mustard (2-3 tbsp.)
- Onion (1, chopped)
- Salt and pepper (to taste)
- Apples (2, chunked)
- Extra-virgin olive oil (2 tbsp.)
- Chicken thighs (8)

How it is done:
- Before you start, make sure to set your oven to 450F.
- Place chicken into a heated pan with olive oil and let it cook until it reaches a golden brown color, which would be around 6 minutes. Once it has reached that state, turn it over and let it cook for another 3 minutes, then put on a plate.
- In the same pan or baking dish, place the onion and apples and use salt and pepper to flavor. Allow them to stay in the pan for around 4 minutes. While this is happening, take your mustard and broth and combine the two, then pour it into the skillet as well, allowing it to boil.
- Put the chicken back into the skillet and then place it in the oven for 18-20 minutes.
- Once the time is done, you should have a butter and flour mixture made up and ready to be mixed into the juices in the skillet left over after you remove the chicken, onion, and apples. Try to make the

consistency into a thick liquid.
- Pour over the chicken and serve.

Creamy Lemon-Pepper Orzo with Grilled Chicken

For this dish, you can expect to produce 4 servings, with an estimated time of around 15 minutes for any preparation, along with around 35 minutes of cooking or baking the ingredients.

Each serving includes:

9.5 g Fat

21 g Protein

37 g Carbohydrates

What is in it:
- Chopped basil (4 tbsp.)
- Goat cheese (2 oz.)
- Chicken thighs, boneless skinless (3)
- Frozen peas (1 cup)
- Orzo Whole-wheat grain (1 cup)
- Lemon (1, zest and juice)
- Salt and pepper (to your own taste)
- Garlic (1 clove, minced)

- Olive oil (3 tsp.)
- Greek yogurt (.25 cup)

How it is done:
- In order to prepare, get a pot of water boiling and start warming up your grill.
- Mix your lemon juice, yogurt, 2 teaspoons of oil, garlic and .5 teaspoon of salt and pepper together.
- Pour 1 teaspoon of oil onto the chicken and season with salt and pepper, then put it on the grill and cook for 10-12 minutes.
- Place the orzo into the pot and allow it to cook based on the directions on package. Add in the peas during the last minute of cook time.
- Mix in the orzo and peas with the yogurt and goat cheese, then also add in the herbs and .75 cups of the liquid from cooking the orzo.
- Combine with chicken and serve.

Middle Eastern Chicken, Veggies, and Rice

For this dish, you can expect to produce 4 servings, with an estimated time of around 15 minutes for any preparation, along with around 15 minutes of cooking or baking the ingredients.

Each serving includes:

17 g Fat

29 g Protein

57 g Carbohydrates

What is in it:
- Parsley (.25 cup)
- Rotisserie chicken (10 oz.)
- Salt
- Cinnamon (.75 tbsp.)
- Chicken broth (.75 cup)
- Bell pepper (1, sliced)
- White onion (1, diced)
- Grapeseed oil (1 tbsp.)
- Rice (4 cups cooked)
- Green beans (8 oz.)

How it is done:
- Cook your rice by following the directions on the label.
- Use a wok or deep pan to heat up the oil, then place the green beans and onions in and stir for five minutes.
- Place the peppers in with .5 teaspoon of salt and continue cooking for another 3 minutes.
- Pour in the broth.
- Place the chicken, rice, and spice in the wok or skillet

and let it simmer, getting rid of any extra liquid.

Sesame-Lemon Chicken

For this dish, you can expect to produce 4 servings, with an estimated time of around 15 minutes for any preparation, along with around 20 minutes of cooking or baking the ingredients.

Each serving includes:

17 g Fat

30 g Protein

22 g Carbohydrates

What is in it:
- Pita chips (2 cups, crushed)
- Cucumber (1, sliced)
- Romaine lettuce hearts (2, cut)
- Tomato (1, sliced)
- Red wine vinegar (2 tbsp.)
- Chicken thighs (8)
- Olive oil (2 tbsp.)
- Lemon juice (1 tbsp.)
- Thyme (2 tsp.)
- Salt and pepper

- Lemon zest (1 tbsp.)
- Sugar (.5 tsp.)
- Sesame seeds (1 tbsp.)

How it is done:
- Mix together your lemon zest, sugar, sesame seeds, salt, and pepper, then season the chicken with most of it, but leave a little bit left out.
- Broil the chicken for around 8-10 minutes on each side.
- With the spice mix you had left over, mix in vinegar, salt, and lemon juice as well as olive oil. After the chicken has cooked, pour this mixture over the top.
- Add the veggies and chips to the plate and serve.

Roasted Rosemary Chicken

For this dish, you can expect to produce 4 servings, with an estimated time of around 20 minutes for any preparation, along with around 65 minutes of cooking or baking the ingredients.

Each serving includes:

16 g Fat

32 g Protein

27 g Carbohydrates

What is in it:
- Black pepper
- Salt
- Olive oil (1 tbsp.)
- Chicken breast, bone-in (4)
- Rosemary (1.5 tsp.)

How it is done:
- Make sure to heat your oven to 450 F before you being.
- Grab a baking pan and place parchment paper on it.
- Cook the chicken in a skillet with oil, using salt and pepper to season, for around 4-5 minutes on each side.
- Allow the chicken to cook in the oven for another 25-30 minutes after it has cooked on the stove, sprinkling with rosemary before you put it in.
- Remove the chicken, let cool, then serve.

Honey Mustard and Red Onion BBQ Chicken

For this dish, you can expect to produce 4 servings, with an estimated time of around 5 minutes for any preparation, along with around 20 minutes of cooking or baking the ingredients.

Each serving includes:

17 g Fat

55 g Protein

27 g Carbohydrates

What is in it:
- Salt and pepper
- Vegetable oil
- Chicken thighs and breasts, boneless skinless (4 each)
- Allspice (.5 tsp.)
- Chicken stock (1 cup)
- Curry powder (.5 tsp.)
- Honey mustard (.5 cup)apple cider vinegar (.25 cup)
- Red onion (.5, cut)
- Brown sugar (.25 cup)

How it is done:
- Put 2 tablespoons of vegetable oil in a pan and cook onions for 5 minutes, place the vinegar in and cook for 2 minutes, place brown sugar in and cook for another minute. Add broth, curry, mustard, and allspice, and let bubble on low heat.
- Grill chicken for 4-5 on each side. Cover in the sauce

you made then cook another 4-5 minutes.

Crunchy French Onion Chicken

For this dish, you can expect to produce 4 servings, with an estimated time of around 10 minutes for any preparation, along with around 20 minutes of cooking or baking the ingredients.

Each serving includes:

40 g Fat

29 g Protein

32 g Carbohydrates

What is in it:
- Chicken breast, boneless skinless (16 oz.)
- Egg (1)
- French-fried onions (1.3 cups, crunched)

How it is made:
- Make sure to set your oven to 400F before starting.
- Pour onions into a bowl, then also beat the egg in another bowl.

- Place the chicken in the beaten egg, then roll in the onions, making sure to let any looser onion pieces fall off.
- Place the chicken on a baking pan allow it to cook for around 20 minutes, be sure it is 165F before taking it out of the oven.

3 Ingredient Chicken Breasts

For this dish, you can expect to produce 4 servings, with an estimated time of around 10 minutes for any preparation, along with around 30 minutes of cooking or baking the ingredients.

Each serving includes:

14 g Fat

24 g Protein

0 g Carbs

What is in it:
- Chicken breasts, boneless skinless (4, cut in half)
- Salt (1 tsp.)
- Butter (.25 cup)

How it is done:
- Make sure to heat your oven to 350F before you begin baking.
- Melt your butter then mix it with salt.
- Place chicken on a greased baking pan, then cover in the butter mixture.
- Bake the chicken for around 35-45 minutes.
- Serve with a vegetable side.

Fiesta Slow Cooker Shredded Chicken Tacos

For this dish, you can expect to produce 8 servings, with an estimated time of around 10 minutes for any preparation, along with around 6 hours of cooking or baking the ingredients.

Each serving includes:

1.2 g Fat

11.1 g Protein

2.4 g Carbohydrates

What is in it:
- Chicken breast, boneless skinless (16 oz.)
- Taco seasoning (2 tbsp.)

- Chicken broth (1 cup)
- Lettuce (1 head)

How it is made:
- Mix together the chicken broth and taco seasoning.
- Put your chicken breasts into the slow cooker then add the broth mixture over it.
- Cook in the slow cooker for anywhere from 6-8 hours. Once the chicken is done, shred it into smaller bits, then place on top a lettuce leaf, adding whatever toppings you would like to finish.

Simple Roasted Chicken

For this dish, you can expect to produce 6 servings, with an estimated time of around 10 minutes for any preparation, along with around one hour of cooking or baking the ingredients.

Each serving includes:

22.8 g Fat

41 g Protein

2 g Carbohydrates

What is in it:
- Salt

- Lemon (1, sliced)
- Chicken (1 whole, around 4 lbs.)
- Red potatoes (4 oz., cubed)
- Carrots (4, sliced)
- Rosemary (2 tsp.)

How it is done:
- Make sure that your oven is ready to go at 450 F before you begin.
- Put your whole chicken into a large pan for roasting, sprinkling in the potatoes and carrots, as well as the rosemary. Place the lemon into the cavity of the chicken. Salt lightly.
- Allow the chick to cook in the oven until the skin turns brown, which will likely be around an hour. Make sure the temperature of the chicken is 160F if you are unsure.
- Carve the chicken, creating six portions, then store.

Pesto Chicken

For this dish, you can expect to produce 4 servings, with an estimated time of around 10 minutes for any preparation, along with around 25 minutes of cooking or baking the ingredients.

Each serving includes:

19.3 g Fat

31.5 g Protein

2 g Carbohydrates

What is in it:

- Prosciutto (4 slices)
- Basil pesto (.5 cup)
- Chicken breast (4, cut in half)
- Salt and pepper

How it is done:

- Make sure your oven is set to 400F before you begin cooking.
- Place each chicken breast half into a prepared greased baking pan, making sure to spread around 2 tablespoons of pesto onto the breast and wrapping it in a slice of prosciutto before putting it into the pan.
- Place the chicken into the oven for around 25 minutes.
- Remove from the oven and store or serve.

Grilled Chicken Skewers

For this dish, you can expect to produce 8 servings, with an estimated time of around 10 minutes for any preparation, along with around 20 minutes of cooking or baking the ingredients.

Each serving includes:

8 g Fat

26 g Protein

0 g Carbohydrates

What is in it:

- Salt and pepper
- Olive oil (.2 cup)
- Chicken breast, boneless skinless (32 oz., sliced into chunks)

How it is done:

- Make sure your grill is warming up so it is properly heated when the chicken is ready to be cooked.
- On a bamboo skewer, place three chunks of chicken, then drizzle olive oil onto the chicken and season with some salt and pepper.
- Place the skewered chicken onto the grill and cook

for around 7-8 minutes.
- If you would like, grill some tomatoes and peppers as well, then place on the kabob.
- Split into portions then store or serve.

Chicken Quesadilla

For this dish, you can expect to produce 4 servings, with an estimated time of around 10 minutes for any preparation, along with around 15 minutes of cooking or baking the ingredients.

Each serving includes:

27 g Fat

45 g Protein

49 g Carbohydrates

What is in it:

- Chicken breast, skinless boneless (4 cups, shredded)
- Salsa (1 cup)
- Soft shell tortillas (8)
- Pickled jalapeno (1 tsp., chopped)

- Cumin (.25 tsp.)
- Cheddar cheese (.5 cup, shredded)

How it is done:

- Mix together your cumin, chicken, jalapeno, and cheese. With on tortilla already sitting on a pan, place the chicken mixture on top, then flatten it down. Put another tortilla on top, flattening it down again, then cook for around 4 minutes, then flip the tortilla to the other side and cook for another four minutes.
- Serve with salsa and sour cream, or your choice of toppings.

Coconut-Curry Chicken

For this dish, you can expect to produce 4 servings, with an estimated time of around 10 minutes for any preparation, along with around 25 minutes of cooking or baking the ingredients.

Each serving includes:

17 g Fat

36 g Protein

9.4 g Carbohydrates

What is in it:
- Chicken breast, skinless boneless (20 oz.)
- Salt
- Curry powder (2 tsp.)
- Shredded coconut (1 cup)
- Butter (3 tbsp., melted)

How it is made:
- Drizzle our melted butter into a baking pan, making sure that your oven is heated at 350F.
- Mix together the coconut flakes and curry powder, using the butter to coat the chicken first, then dipping it into the coconut mixture.
- Put each piece of chicken onto the baking pan, then season with salt and bake for 20-25 minutes.
- Remove from oven and serve or store the portions, combining with rice and vegetables.

Grilled Chicken and Pineapple Sandwiches

For this dish, you can expect to produce 4 servings, with an estimated time of around 6 minutes for any preparation, along with around 10 minutes of cooking or baking the ingredients.

Each serving includes:

4 g Fat

43.4 g Protein

30.5 Carbohydrates

What is in it:
- Basil leaves (4)
- Light mayo
- Buns (4)
- Pineapple (4 slices)
- Lime juice (.25 cup)
- Pepper (.25 tsp.)
- Salt (.5 tsp.)
- Chicken breast, boneless skinless (4, cut in half)

How it is done:
- Make sure your grill is warmed up and ready to go.
- Use salt and pepper to season your chicken before you cook it.
- Put your chicken onto the grill, cooking for 5-6 minutes on either side. Drizzle lime juice over top of it every so often.
- Place the pineapple onto the grill as well, letting it cook for 2-3 minutes on each side.
- Smear the mayo onto half of the bun, then top with

chicken, pineapple, and a basil leaf.

Vietnamese Stir-Fry

For this dish, you can expect to produce 4 servings, with an estimated time of around 10 minutes for any preparation, along with around 20 minutes of cooking or baking the ingredients.

Each serving includes:

6.2 g Fat

24.4 g Protein

4.7 g Carbohydrates

What is in it:
- Soy sauce (.25 cup)
- Salt (.25 tsp.)
- Chicken breast, boneless skinless (16 oz, diced)
- Sambal oelek (1.5 tbsp.)
- Lemongrass (.3 cup)
- Canola oil 1 tbsp.)

How it is done:
- In an oiled and heated pan, place the lemongrass and

cook it for one minute, making sure to stir it often. Once the time has passed, add the chicken into the pan as well, salting as needed.
- Let both the lemongrass and chicken cook for another 3 minutes.
- Pour the sambal to the chicken pan, cooking for 30 seconds and stirring often.
- Pour the soy sauce in and let the mixture reach a boil. Turn the heat down once it does, then let the mixture simmer for another 5 minutes.
- Split the final product into 4 portions.

Slow Cooker Buffalo Chicken Lettuce Wraps

For this dish, you can expect to produce 10 servings, with an estimated time of around 10 minutes for any preparation, along with around 6 hours of cooking or baking the ingredients.

Each serving includes:

2 g Fat

18 g Protein

2.4 g Carbohydrates

What is in it:
- Lettuce (1 head)
- Ranch dressing mix (1 package)
- Hot sauce (12 oz.)
- Chicken breast, skinless boneless (32 oz.)

How it is done:
- Place your chicken in a slow cooker and allow to sit and cook on the low setting for around 6-7 hours.
- Mix the hot sauce and ranch dressing mix together, then pour over the chicken as it begins to cook.
- Once the time has passed, take the chicken out and shred it up using forks.
- Use the liquid left over from the cooked chicken as a side sauce.
- Place the shredded chicken onto the lettuce leaves and serve or store.

Chapter 3: Beef and Pork

Beef and pork are both staples in many diets, but a little harder to incorporate into healthy recipes. Both are best in moderation if you are trying to be little leaner, but when you do treat yourself to some heartier meats, or if you are looking to bulk up, then the recipes in this chapter will detail a few choices for easy, simple and flavorful beef and pork options.

Brussel Sprouts and Sausage

For this dish, you can expect to produce 4 servings, with an estimated time of around 10 minutes for any preparation, along with around 20 minutes of cooking or baking the ingredients.

Each serving includes around:

14 g Fat

8 g Protein

16 g Carbohydrates

What is in it:
- Salt and pepper
- Water (.5 cup)
- Brussel sprouts (1.5 lbs., cut and trimmed)
- Italian sausage (3.3 oz.)
- Olive oil (2 tbsp.)

How it is done:

- Cook your sausage in a pan with oil, making sure to stir every so often, for around 5 minutes.
- Place Brussel sprouts in the pan as well, then place the water as well as salt and pepper. Cook for around ten more minutes and cover.
- Take the cover off after ten minutes and cook for a few more minutes until the sprouts turn browner, then remove from heat.
- Separate and serve.

Dijon-Brown Sugar Steak

For this dish, you can expect to produce 3 servings, with an estimated time of around 3 hours for any preparation, along with around 15 minutes of cooking or baking the ingredients.

Each serving includes around:

16 g Fat

22 g Protein

1 g Carbohydrates

What is in it:

- Salt and pepper
- Brown sugar (2 tbsp.)
- Dijon mustard (2 tbsp.)
- Olive oil (1 tbsp.)
- Steak (1 lb.)

How it is done:

- Mix oil, salt and pepper, and brown sugar together, then rub the mixture into your steak and let it sit for anywhere from one to four hours in time.
- Once the steak has sat, then place it on the grill and cook it for around 8 minutes, or however long it takes to reach your preferred level of doneness.

Easy 3 Ingredient Chili

For this dish, you can expect to produce 4-6 servings, with an estimated time of around 20 minutes for any preparation, along with around 1-6 of cooking or baking the ingredients.

Each serving includes around:

14 g Fat

29 g Protein

22 g Carbohydrates

What is in it:
- Diced tomatoes (1 can)
- Chili beans (1 can)
- Ground beef (1 lb.)

How it is made:
- Once you have placed your ground beef into a pan and allowed it to brown properly, mix the beans and tomatoes with the cooked meat. Allow the mixture to reach a boil, then let it simmer for another 30 minutes.
- If you prefer to slow cook the chili, then place the mixture into a Crock-Pot and cook it on the lowest setting for anywhere from 4-6 hours.
- Top the chili with your choice of toppings, including sour cream and cheese. Portion out and store the rest.

Grilled PB & B&B Sandwich

For this dish, you can expect to produce 4 servings, with an estimated time of around 10 minutes for any preparation, along with around 10 minutes of cooking or baking the ingredients.

What is in it:

- Banana (2, sliced)
- Bacon (16 strips)
- Peanut butter (8 tbsp.)
- Bread (8 slices, sourdough is recommended)

How it is done:

- Cook your bacon on a griddle until crispy and brown.
- Coat one piece of bread for each sandwich with peanut butter, the place 4 slices of the bacon onto the slice of peanut butter break. Place the banana slices on top of that, then top with the second piece of bread.
- Using the leftover bacon fat, grill the completed sandwiches until they are golden.
- Serve and store the rest.

Cajun Dijon Grilled Pork Tenderloin

For this dish, you can expect to produce 4-6 servings, with an estimated time of around 10 minutes for any preparation, along with around one hour of cooking or baking the ingredients.

Each serving includes around:

5 g Fat

26 g Protein

0 g Carbohydrates

What is in it:

- Pork tenderloin (1.5 lbs.)
- Cajun seasoning (3 tbsp.)
- Orange (1)
- Dijon mustard (1 cup)

How it is done:

- Mix the mustard, the juice from the orange, and the Cajun seasoning together.
- In a bag, put the pork and seasoning mix together and allow the pork to sit in the mix in the fridge for around 30 minutes.

- Once the time has passed, grill the pork for around 10-12 minutes on both sides.
- Separate the finished pork into portions and serve with rice and veggies.

Mexican Stuffed Peppers

For this dish, you can expect to produce 8 servings, with an estimated time of around 25 minutes for any preparation, along with around 30 minutes of cooking or baking the ingredients.

Each serving includes:

9 g Fat

19 g Protein

26 g Carbohydrates

What is in it:
- Mexican cheese blend (2 cups, shredded)
- Sweet peppers (8)
- Waer (1.5 cups)
- Mexican Rice and pasta mix (1 packet)
- Diced tomatoes (1 can)
- Ground beef (1 lb.)

How it is done:

- Make sure your oven is ready to go at 375F.
- Brown the ground beef in a pan, then drain the excess grease off.
- Add the tomatoes, rice mix and water to the beef, then allow the mix to boil, turning the heat down once it does and letting it simmer for around 8 minutes.
- Cut the tops off of the peppers and remove the insides, the scoop .3 cups of the beef into the peppers and sprinkle with cheese. The rest of the topping should be the rice mix.
- Place the peppers into the oven and cook for 25 minutes.
- Remove from the oven and put the rest of the cheese over the top, putting it back in the oven for another 5 minutes so the cheese melts.
- Serve and separate into portions.

Asian Meatballs

For this dish, you can expect to produce 6 servings, with an estimated time of around 25 minutes for any preparation, along with around 50 minutes of cooking or baking the ingredients.

Each serving includes:

9 g Fat

18 g Protein

13 g Carbohydrates

What is in it:
- Ground beef (1 lb.)
- Pepper (.5 tsp.)
- Salt (.5 tsp.)
- Ginger (1 tbsp., chopped)
- Dry sherry (2 tbsp.)
- Scallions (.25 cup, chopped)
- Water chestnuts (8 oz., diced)
- Olive oil (1 tbsp.)
- Breadcrumbs (.5 cup)
- Garlic (4 cloves, minced)
- Celery (1 stalk)
- Onion (1, diced)
- Mushrooms (8 oz., diced)

How it is done:
- Place the garlic, celery, mushrooms, and onions into a food processor and process them until they are finely chopped. Place them in a heated pan with oil and cook for 6-8 minutes, stirring every so often. Once done, take off the burner and allow it to sit and cool for around 10 minutes.

- Make sure your oven is warming up and ready to go at 450F.
- Place the scallions, breadcrumbs, sherry, water chestnuts, ginger, salt, and pepper with the cooled vegetable mix and stir them together. Also, add the beef to the mix and continue stirring.
- Ball the mixture into meatball sized portions, then put them on a greased baking pan.
- Place the meatballs into the oven for around 15 minutes.
- Remove and serve, then portion out the rest.

Porcupine Meatballs

For this dish, you can expect to produce 6 servings, with an estimated time of around 30 minutes for any preparation, along with around 2 ¾
hours of cooking or baking the ingredients.

Each serving includes:

1 g Fat

4 g Protein

27 g Carbohydrates

What is in it:

- Ground beef (1.5 lbs.)
- Pepper (.25 tsp.)
- Salt (.5 tsp.)
- Garlic powder (.5 tsp.)
- Onion powder (1 tsp.)
- Dried thyme (1 tsp.)
- Onion (.25 cup, diced)
- Rice (.75 cup, white or brown)
- Hot sauce (2 tsp.)
- Worcestershire sauce (1 tbsp.)
- Water (2 cups)
- Tomato sauce (28 oz.)

How it is done:
- Make sure your oven is warming up and ready to go at 350 F.
- Mix together the water, hot sauce, tomato sauce, and Worcestershire sauce in a Dutch oven.
- In a bowl, mix the rice, onion powder, onion, garlic powder, thyme, salt, and pepper together. Add in the ground beef, then continue mixing.
- Form the beef into meatball sizes and add them in with the sauce mixture.
- Allow the meatballs to bake for around 2 hours covered, cooking rice while the meatballs are almost done.
- Once finished, serve the meatballs over rice and store the rest of the portions.

Stuffed Tomatoes

For this dish, you can expect to produce 4 servings, with an estimated time of around 10 minutes for any preparation, along with around 6 hours of cooking or baking the ingredients.

Each serving contains:

16 g Fat

21 g Protein

33 g Carbohydrates

What is in it:
- Breadcrumbs (1 cup)
- Garlic (1 clove, minced)
- Green peas (.5 cup)
- Parmesan (.5 cup)
- Olive oil (2 tbsp.)
- Parsley (1 tbsp.)
- Salt (.5 tsp.)
- Red onion (.25 cup)
- Pepper
- Brown rice (.5 cup)
- Ground beef (4 oz.)

- Tomatoes (4)

How it is done:
- Make sure your oven is warming up and ready to go at 350F.
- Brown the ground beef.
- Cook up the rice that you choose by following the package directions.
- Place the rice and meat in the same bowl.
- Cut off the tomato tops, then scoop the insides out using a spoon. Take out .5 cup of the pulp and add it to the rice and meat mix, along with peas, onion, .25 cup of cheese and parsley.
- Salt and pepper the mixture to your own taste then stir it all together.
- Scoop out the mixture and place it into the tomatoes as evenly as possible, then sprinkle the rest of the cheese along with breadcrumbs on top of the tomatoes.
- Place the tomatoes into the oven and allow them to cook for around 25-30 minutes.

Mini Meatloaves with Green Beans and Potatoes

For this dish, you can expect to produce 4 servings, with an estimated time of around 20 minutes for any preparation, along with around 40 minutes of cooking or baking the ingredients.

Each serving includes:

20 g Fat

29 g Protein

36 g Carbohydrates

What is in it:
- Green beans (1 lb.)
- Worcestershire sauce (1 tbsp.)
- Onion (.25 cup, diced)
- Ketchup (3 tbsp.)
- Egg (1)
- Italian panko breadcrumbs (.25 cup)
- Olive oil (2 tbsp.)
- Pepper (.75 tsp.)
- Ground beef (1 lb.)
- Salt (.75 tsp.)
- Garlic powder (.5 tsp.)
- Paprika (.5 tsp.)
- Potatoes (1 lb.)

How it is done:
- Make sure your oven is warming up and ready to go

at 425F.
- Mix the paprika and half the garlic powder together with some salt and pepper. Spread over the potatoes along with some olive oil then place them in the oven to roast for ten minutes.
- Mix the beef, egg, 2/3 of the ketchup, salt, and pepper, breadcrumbs, Worcestershire sauce, and onion together, then mold it into four mini-sized loaves. Place the loaves onto a baking sheet and coat the tops with the other 1/3 of ketchup, then place in the oven for around 40 minutes.
- Mix the green beans with 1 tablespoon of oil and salt and pepper, then add them to the same pan as the potatoes, putting them back into the oven for another 20-30 minutes.

Chapter 4: Breakfast Recipes

Though there is not a ton of space left to over breakfast meals, the most important meal of the day still deserves its turn in the cookbook spotlight. Prepping breakfast is one of the most efficient choices you can make, as in the grand scheme of things, breakfast is often the easiest meal to forget. By planning ahead and portioning out some of these recipes, you free yourself up to do whatever you would like with your extra time in the morning, whether that be sleeping in a little longer or getting a head start on the morning traffic. You can't go wrong when it comes to planning ahead in the morning, and these recipes will help you out with that.

Brie and Cranberry Phyllo Turnovers

For this dish, you can expect to produce 7-9 servings, with an estimated time of around 25 minutes for any preparation, along with around 10 minutes of cooking or baking the ingredients.

Each serving includes:

2 g Fat

2 g Protein

4 g Carbohydrates

What is in it:
- Cranberry sauce (2 tbsp.)
- Brie (3 oz.)
- Filo dough (1 roll, .5 packages)

How it is done:
- Make sure your oven is warming up and ready to go at 375 F.
- Take out the dough and unroll it, then place the dough on a greased cooking pan, placing two more layers on top and greasing each.
- Slice the dough into sections of three and put one piece of Brie and .5 teaspoons of cranberry sauce inside the dough, leaving about .75 inches of a gap at the ends of the dough.
- Fold the dough up into a crescent shape, the place on another baking pan that is not greased.
- Put the dough pockets into the oven for around 12-15 minutes.

Paleo Pancakes

For this dish, you can expect to produce 8 servings, with an estimated time of around 5 minutes for any preparation, along with around 15 minutes of cooking or baking the ingredients.

What is in it:
- Coconut oil
- Coconut flour (.3 cup)
- Eggs (6)
- Bananas (3)

How it is done:
- Blend the coconut flour, bananas, eggs, and a dash of salt until it reaches a smooth consistency. Once smoothed out, place the batter in dollops into a pan greased with the coconut oil, then cook each pancake until it reaches the brownness level you desire.
- Serve and store the rest.

Chia Pudding

For this dish, you can expect to produce 4 servings, with an estimated time of around 5 minutes for any preparation, along with around 5 minutes of cooking or baking the ingredients.

What is in it:
- Maple syrup (.25 cup)
- Vanilla (.5 tsp.)
- Chia seeds (.5 cup)
- Coconut milk (2 cups)

How it is done:
- Place all of the ingredients except for the chia seeds into a blender and blend until it reaches a smooth consistency. Mix in the chia seeds after.
- Place the mix into jars and keep in fridge until ready to serve.

Chocolate Chip Oatmeal Breakfast Cookie

For this dish, you can expect to produce 8-10 servings, with an estimated time of around 10 minutes for any preparation, along with around 15 minutes of cooking or baking the ingredients.

Each serving includes:

3 g Fat

2 g Protein

19 g Carbohydrates

What is in it:
- Chocolate chips (.25 cups)
- Oats (1 cup)
- Bananas (2, mashed)

How it is done:
- Make sure your oven is warming up and ready to go at 350 F.
- Mix the bananas and oats together, then slowly fold in the chocolate chips to the mixture. Place dollops of the mix onto a greased baking pan.
- Allow the cookies to bake in the oven for around 15 minutes, then remove and let cool.
- Serve and store the rest.

Cheddar Broccoli Egg Muffin

For this dish, you can expect to produce 6 servings, with an estimated time of around 10 minutes for any preparation, along with around 15 minutes of cooking or baking the ingredients.

What is in it:
- Salt and pepper
- Cheddar cheese (.5 cup, grated)

- Steamed broccoli (1 cup)
- Eggs (4)

How it is done:
- Make sure your oven is warming up and ready to go at 375F.
- Cut up the broccoli and mix it with eggs and salt and pepper if desired.
- Using muffin tins, pour in the eggs and place the mixture into the oven and allow it to bake for 14-15 minutes.
- Remove from the oven, let cool, serve, and store the rest.

Almond Butter Granola Bars

For this dish, you can expect to produce 8-10 servings, with an estimated time of around 10 minutes for any preparation, along with around 15 minutes of cooking or baking the ingredients.

What is in it:
- Oats (3 cups)
- Almond butter (1 cup)
- Honey (.75 cup)

How it is done:
- Make sure your oven is warming up and ready to go at 350 F.
- In a pan, allow the almond butter and honey to heat and melt, stirring occasionally then take off of the stove once melted.
- Drizzle this mixture over the oats and stir them together well.
- Put the combined mixture on a baking sheet and cook for 15 minutes.
- Serve and store the rest.

Flourless Peanut Butter Muffins

For this dish, you can expect to produce 6-8 servings, with an estimated time of around 5 minutes for any preparation, along with around 20 minutes of cooking or baking the ingredients.

What is in it:
- Sea salt
- Dates (6, pitted)
- Peanut butter (1 cup)
- Bananas (2)

How it is done:
- Make sure your oven is warming up and ready to go at 350 F.
- Put the ingredients into a food processor or blender and mix until smooth.
- Place the mixture into a greased muffin pan, then place the muffins into the oven and allow them to bake for around 15-20 minutes.
- Once cool, remove the muffins, serve and store the rest for later.

Ham, Kale, Cauliflower, and Egg Muffins

For this dish, you can expect to produce 6 servings, with an estimated time of around 10 minutes for any preparation, along with around 20 minutes of cooking or baking the ingredients.

Each serving includes:

4.3 g Fat
7 g Protein
2.8 g Carbohydrates

What is in it:
- Cauliflower (1 cup)
- Salt and pepper
- Ham (.75 cup)

- Kale (1 cup)
- Eggs (3)

How it is done:
- Make sure your oven is warming up and ready to go at 400F.
- Use a food processor or blender to make the cauliflower into a rice-like consistency.
- Mix the eggs together with the cauliflower rice, kale, and ham, then add salt and pepper.
- Pour the mix into greased muffin tins and cook for 20 minutes.

Fruit and Yogurt Cups

For this dish, you can expect to produce 4-6 servings, with an estimated time of around 10 minutes for any preparation, along with around zero minutes of cooking or baking the ingredients.

What is in it:
- Fruit of your choice, including berries, kiwi, oranges, cherries, mango and apples (1.25 cups, chopped)
- Yogurt of your choice (1.5 cups)
- Jars (8 oz.)

How it is done:
- Place fruit at the bottom of the jar as a base, just a few tablespoons.
- Add yogurt to the jar next, then layer with more

fruit.
- Feel free to choose the number of layers you add in, as well as any other toppings.
- Store the cups and top with granola, honey, etc when served.

Breakfast Taquitos

For this dish, you can expect to produce 10-15 servings, with an estimated time of around 10 minutes for any preparation, along with around 30 minutes of cooking or baking the ingredients.

Each serving includes:

19.5 g Fat

30 g Protein

27.5 g Carbohydrates

What is in it:
- Tortillas (20)
- Cilantro (.3 cup, sliced)
- Red onion (1, chopped)
- Cheddar cheese (1 cup, grated)
- Bell pepper (1, diced)
- Sweet potato (.5, diced)

- Olive oil (3 tbsp.)
- Eggs (10)
- Sausage (1 lb.)
- Fennel seeds (1 tbsp.)

How it is done:
- Make sure your oven is warming up and ready to go at 350 F.
- Cook your sweet potatoes in a heated pan with oil for around 10 minutes, then throw in the onion and peppers as well, allowing the mixture to cook for 4 more minutes. Remove from the stove.
- Cook the sausage over the stove, adding in the fennel seeds for seasoning.
- Whip the eggs together and scramble them up.
- Put the tortillas in a baking pan and fill them up with cheese, egg, sausage, and vegetable mix, topping with a little bit of cilantro
- Allow the taquitos to cook in the oven for around 10 minutes total, then remove them, serve, and freeze the rest.

Meal prep recipes

Italian Veggie Salad

Total Time
Prep: 30 min. + chilling
Makes
16 servings
Ingredients
- 2 cups fresh baby carrots, quartered lengthwise
- 1-3/4 cups thinly sliced radishes
- 2 celery ribs, sliced
- 1 small head cauliflower, broken into florets
- 1 bunch broccoli, cut into florets
- 6 large fresh mushrooms, thinly sliced
- 1 can (2-1/4 ounces) sliced ripe olives, drained
- 1 package Italian salad dressing mix
- 1/3 cup water
- 1/3 cup white vinegar
- 1/3 cup olive oil
- 1 package (9 ounces) hearts of romaine salad mix

Pepperoncini, optional

Directions

1. In a large bowl, combine the first seven ingredients. In a small bowl, whisk the dressing mix, water, vinegar and oil. Pour over vegetables; toss to coat. Cover and refrigerate for at least 4 hours.
2. Just before serving, place romaine in a large serving bowl. Add vegetables; toss to coat. Top with pepperoncini if desired.

Nutrition Facts
1 cup: 75 calories, 5g fat (1g saturated fat), 0 cholesterol, 237mg sodium, 6g carbohydrate (3g sugars, 3g fiber), 2g protein. Diabetic Exchanges: 1 vegetable, 1 fat.

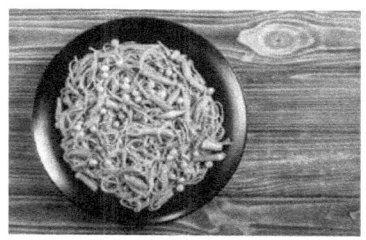

Edamame and Soba Noodle Bowl

Total Time
Prep/Total Time: 30 min.
Makes
6 servings
Ingredients
- 1 package (12 ounces) uncooked Japanese soba noodles or whole wheat spaghetti
- 2 tablespoons sesame oil
- 2 cups fresh small broccoli florets
- 1 medium onion, halved and thinly sliced
- 3 cups frozen shelled edamame, thawed
- 2 large carrots, cut into ribbons with a vegetable peeler
- 4 garlic cloves, minced

- 1 cup reduced-fat Asian toasted sesame salad dressing
- 1/4 teaspoon pepper

Sesame seeds, toasted, optional

Directions

1. In a 6 qt. stockpot, cook noodles according to package directions; drain and return to pan.
2. Meanwhile, in a large skillet, heat oil over medium heat. Add broccoli and onion; cook and stir until crisp-tender, 4-6 minutes. Add edamame and carrots; cook and stir until tender, 6-8 minutes. Add garlic; cook 1 minute longer. Add vegetable mixture, dressing and pepper to noodles; toss to combine. Sprinkle with sesame seeds if desired.

Nutrition Facts

1-1/3 cups: 414 calories, 12g fat (1g saturated fat), 0 cholesterol, 867mg sodium, 64g carbohydrate (12g sugars, 4g fiber), 18g protein.

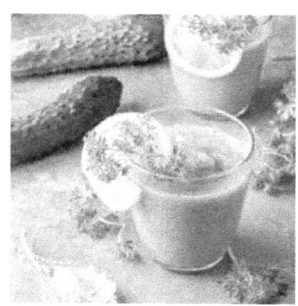

Cucumber, Lemon, and Sage Sipper

Prep Time: 5 minutes
Total Time: 5 minutes
Servings: 2 servings
Ingredients
- 1 cup ice
- 2 cups sparkling water (tap water would be fine)
- 2 cups cucumber
- 1/2 cup lemon juice
- 1 teaspoon lemon rind
- 2 tablespoons sage (finely chopped)

2 teaspoons sweetener of choice (optional)
Instructions
1. Combine all ingredients in blender and blend until well mixed. Serve over ice and garnish with cucumber or lemon slices and a sprig of sage.

Nutrition
Calories: 36kcal | Carbohydrates: 8g | Protein: 1g | Sodium: 103mg | Potassium: 265mg | Fiber: 1g | Sugar: 3g | Vitamin A: 215IU | Vitamin C: 29.8mg | Calcium: 75mg | Iron: 0.9mg

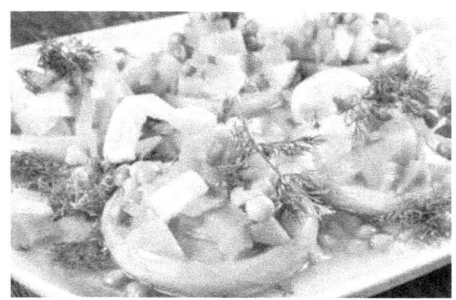

Vegan Lentils with Kale Artichoke Saute

Total Time
Prep/Total Time: 30 min.
Makes
4 servings
Ingredients
- 1/2 cup dried red lentils, rinsed and sorted
- 1/4 teaspoon dried oregano
- 1/8 teaspoon pepper
- 1-1/4 cups vegetable broth
- 1/4 teaspoon sea salt, divided
- 1 tablespoon olive oil or grapeseed oil
- 16 cups chopped fresh kale (about 12 ounces)
- 1 can (14 ounces) water-packed artichoke hearts, drained and chopped
- 3 garlic cloves, minced
- 1/2 teaspoon Italian seasoning
- 2 tablespoons grated Romano cheese (or vegan replacement)

2 cups hot cooked brown or basmati rice

Directions
1. Place first 4 ingredients and 1/8 teaspoon salt in a small saucepan; bring to a boil. Reduce heat; simmer, covered, until lentils are tender and liquid is almost absorbed, 12-15 minutes. Remove from heat.
2. In a 6-qt. stockpot, heat oil over medium heat. Add kale and remaining salt; cook, covered, until kale is wilted, 4-5 minutes, stirring occasionally. Add artichoke hearts, garlic and Italian seasoning; cook and stir 3 minutes. Remove from heat; stir in cheese.
3. Serve lentils and kale mixture over rice.

Nutrition Facts
1 serving: 321 calories, 6g fat (2g saturated fat), 1mg cholesterol, 661mg sodium, 53g carbohydrate (1g sugars, 5g fiber), 15g protein.

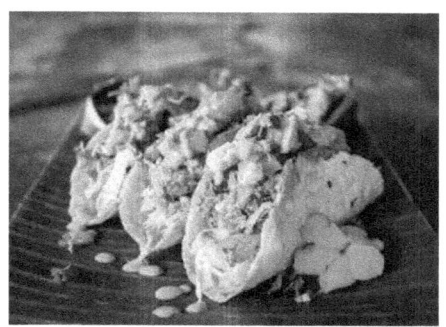

Vegan Taco Appetizers

Total Time
Prep: 25 min. + chilling
Makes
about 5 dozen
Ingredients
- 1 package (8 ounces) cream cheese (or vegan replacement), softened
- 1 tablespoon taco seasoning
- 1 can (16 ounces) refried beans
- 8 flour tortillas (10 inches), room temperature
- 3 cups shredded lettuce
- 2 large tomatoes, seeded and finely chopped
- 2 cans (4 ounces each) chopped green chilies
- 1 cup finely chopped ripe olives

Salsa

Directions
1. In a small bowl, beat cream cheese and taco seasoning until blended. Stir in the refried beans. Spread 3-4 tablespoons over each tortilla. Layer

lettuce, tomatoes, chilies and olives down the center of each tortilla; roll up tightly to 2-in. diameter.
2. Wrap in plastic and refrigerate for at least 1 hour. Cut into 1-in. slices. Serve with salsa.

Nutrition Facts
1 each: 54 calories, 2g fat (1g saturated fat), 5mg cholesterol, 135mg sodium, 6g carbohydrate (0 sugars, 1g fiber), 2g protein. Diabetic Exchanges: 1/2 starch, 1/2 fat.

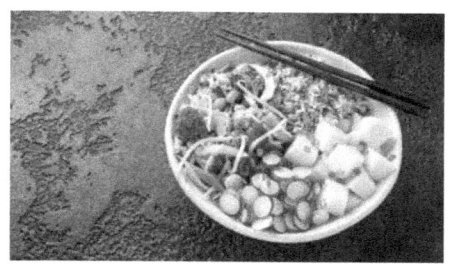

Veggie-Cashew Stir-Fry

Total Time
Prep: 20 min. Cook: 15 min.
Makes
4 servings
Ingredients
- 1/4 cup reduced-sodium soy sauce
- 1/4 cup water
- 2 tablespoons brown sugar
- 2 tablespoons lemon juice
- 2 tablespoons olive oil
- 1 garlic clove, minced
- 2 cups sliced fresh mushrooms
- 1/4 pound fresh baby carrots, coarsely chopped
- 1 small zucchini, cut into 1/4-inch slices
- 1 small sweet red pepper, coarsely chopped
- 1 small green pepper, coarsely chopped
- 4 green onions, sliced
- 2 cups cooked brown rice
- 1 can (8 ounces) sliced water chestnuts, drained

1/2 cup honey-roasted cashews

Directions
1. In a small bowl, mix soy sauce, water, brown sugar and lemon juice until smooth; set aside.
2. In a large skillet, heat oil over medium-high heat. Stir-fry garlic for 1 minute. Add vegetables; cook until vegetables are crisp-tender, 6-8 minutes.
3. Stir soy sauce mixture and add to pan. Bring to a boil. Add rice and water chestnuts; heat through. Top with cashews.

Nutrition Facts
1-1/2 cups: 385 calories, 16g fat (3g saturated fat), 0 cholesterol, 671mg sodium, 56g carbohydrate (15g sugars, 6g fiber), 9g protein.

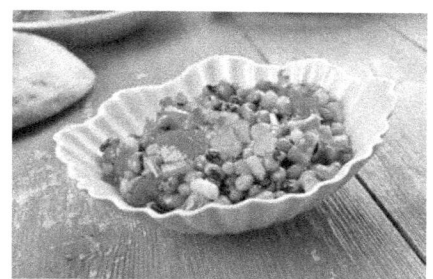

Vibrant Black-Eyed Pea Salad

Total Time
Prep: 25 min. + chilling
Makes
10 servings
Ingredients
- 2 cans (15-1/2 ounces each) black-eyed peas, rinsed and drained
- 2 cups grape tomatoes, halved
- 1 each small green, yellow and red peppers, finely chopped
- 1 small red onion, chopped
- 1 celery rib, chopped

2 tablespoons minced fresh basil
DRESSING:
- 1/4 cup red wine vinegar or balsamic vinegar
- 1 tablespoon stone-ground mustard
- 1 teaspoon minced fresh oregano or 1/4 teaspoon dried oregano
- 3/4 teaspoon salt
- 1/2 teaspoon freshly ground pepper

1/4 cup olive oil

Directions

1. In a large bowl, combine peas, tomatoes, peppers, onion, celery and basil.
2. For dressing, in a small bowl, whisk vinegar, mustard, oregano, salt and pepper. Gradually whisk in oil until blended. Drizzle over salad; toss to coat. Refrigerate, covered, at least 3 hours before serving.

Nutrition Facts
3/4 cup: 130 calories, 6g fat (1g saturated fat), 0 cholesterol, 319mg sodium, 15g carbohydrate (3g sugars, 3g fiber), 5g protein. Diabetic exchanges: 1 starch, 1 fat.

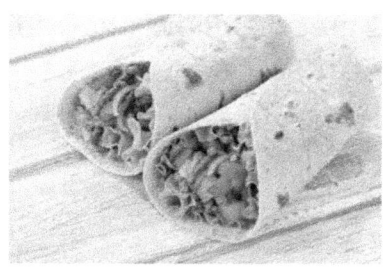

Quick Taco Wraps

Total Time
Prep/Total Time: 15 min.
Makes
4 servings

Ingredients
- 1/2 cup cream cheese (or vegan replacement), softened
- 1/4 cup canned chopped green chilies
- 1/4 cup sour cream
- 2 tablespoons taco seasoning
- 1/2 cup bean dip
- 4 flour tortillas (10 inches)
- 1/2 cup guacamole dip
- 1 small onion, chopped
- 1 small sweet red pepper, chopped
- 1/2 cup shredded cheddar cheese

1 can (2-1/4 ounces) sliced ripe olives, drained

Directions
1. In a small bowl, beat cream cheese until smooth. Stir in green chilies, sour cream and taco seasoning.
2. Spread bean dip over tortillas to within 1/2 in. of edges. Layer with guacamole dip, cream cheese mixture, onion, pepper, cheese and olives. Roll up tightly and serve.

Nutrition Facts
1 wrap: 533 calories, 28g fat (13g saturated fat), 51mg cholesterol, 1538mg sodium, 48g carbohydrate (3g sugars, 8g fiber), 14g protein.

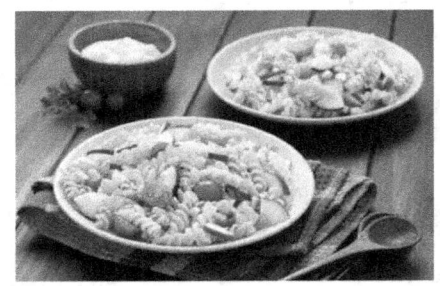

Colorful Spiral Pasta Salad

Total Time
Prep/Total Time: 20 min.
Makes
14 servings
Ingredients
- 1 package (12 ounces) tricolor spiral pasta
- 4 cups fresh broccoli florets
- 1 pint grape tomatoes
- 1 can (6 ounces) pitted ripe olives, drained
- 1/8 teaspoon salt
- 1/8 teaspoon pepper

1-1/2 cups Italian salad dressing with roasted red pepper and Parmesan

Directions

1. In a Dutch oven, cook pasta according to package directions, adding the broccoli during the last 2 minutes of cooking. Drain and rinse in cold water.
2. Transfer to a large bowl. Add the tomatoes, olives, salt and pepper. Drizzle with salad dressing; toss to coat. Chill until serving.

Nutrition Facts
3/4 cup: 149 calories, 4g fat (0 saturated fat), 0 cholesterol, 513mg sodium, 24g carbohydrate (4g sugars, 2g fiber), 4g protein.

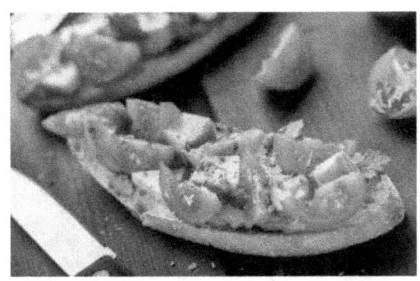

Avocado Bruschetta

Total Time
Prep/Total Time: 20 min.
Makes
2 dozen
Ingredients
- 1/2 cup olive oil
- 1/4 cup lemon juice
- 1/4 cup red wine vinegar
- 3 garlic cloves, minced
- 1-1/2 teaspoons salt
- 1 teaspoon crushed red pepper flakes
- 1 teaspoon dried oregano
- 1/2 teaspoon pepper
- 1/2 cup chopped fresh cilantro
- 1/2 cup chopped fresh parsley
- 1/4 cup chopped fresh basil
- 6 medium ripe avocados, peeled and cubed

24 slices French bread baguette (1/2 inch thick)
Directions

1. Preheat broiler. Whisk together first 8 ingredients; stir in herbs. Fold in avocados. Place bread on an ungreased baking sheet. Broil 3-4 in. from heat until golden brown, 1-2 minutes per side. Top with avocado mixture.

Nutrition Facts
1 appetizer: 118 calories, 10g fat (1g saturated fat), 0 cholesterol, 199mg sodium, 8g carbohydrate (0 sugars, 2g fiber), 2g protein

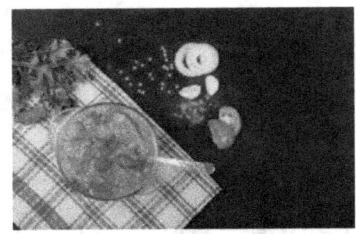

Tomato-Garlic Lentil Bowls

Total Time
Prep/Total Time: 30 min.
Makes
6 servings
Ingredients
- 1 tablespoon olive oil
- 2 medium onions, chopped
- 4 garlic cloves, minced
- 2 cups dried brown lentils, rinsed
- 1 teaspoon salt
- 1/2 teaspoon ground ginger
- 1/2 teaspoon paprika
- 1/4 teaspoon pepper
- 3 cups water
- 1/4 cup lemon juice
- 3 tablespoons tomato paste
- 3/4 cup fat-free plain Greek yogurt

Optional: Chopped tomatoes and minced fresh cilantro
Directions
1. In a large saucepan, heat oil over medium-high heat; saute onions 2 minutes. Add garlic; cook 1

minute. Stir in lentils, seasonings and water; bring to a boil. Reduce heat; simmer, covered, until lentils are tender, 25-30 minutes.
2. Stir in lemon juice and tomato paste; heat through. Serve with yogurt and, if desired, tomatoes and cilantro.
3. Health Tip: Cup for cup, lentils have twice as much protein and iron as ?uinoa.

Nutrition Facts
3/4 cup: 294 calories, 3g fat (0 saturated fat), 0 cholesterol, 419mg sodium, 49g carbohydrate (5g sugars, 8g fiber), 21g protein. Diabetic exchanges: 3 starch, 2 lean meat, 1/2 fat

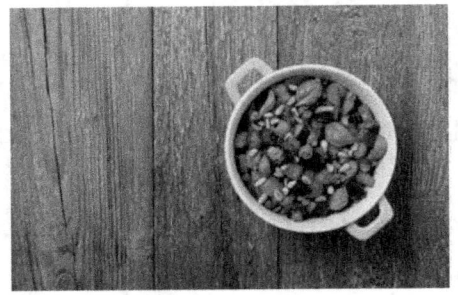

Pressure-Cooker Caponata

Total Time
Prep: 20 min. Cook: 5 min.
Makes
6 cups
Ingredients
- 2 medium eggplants, cut into 1/2-inch pieces
- 1 can (14-1/2 ounces) diced tomatoes, undrained
- 1 medium onion, chopped
- 1/2 cup dry red wine
- 12 garlic cloves, sliced
- 3 tablespoons extra virgin olive oil
- 2 tablespoons red wine vinegar
- 4 teaspoons capers, undrained
- 5 bay leaves
- 1-1/2 teaspoons salt
- 1/4 teaspoon coarsely ground pepper
- French bread baguette slices, toasted

Optional toppings: Fresh basil leaves, toasted pine nuts and additional olive oil
Directions

1. Place the first 11 ingredients in a 6-qt. electric pressure cooker (do not stir). Lock lid; close pressure-release valve. Adjust to pressure-cook on high for 3 minutes. Quick-release pressure.
2. Cool slightly; discard bay leaves. Serve with toasted baguette slices. If desired, serve with toppings.

Nutrition Facts
1/4 cup: 34 calories, 2g fat (0 saturated fat), 0 cholesterol, 189mg sodium, 5g carbohydrate (2g sugars, 2g fiber), 1g protein.

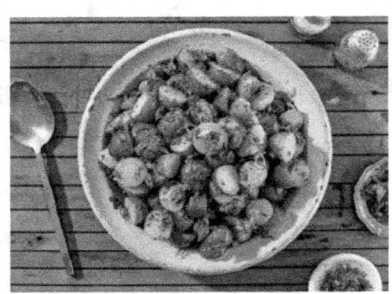

Herb-Vinaigrette Potato Salad

Total Time
Prep: 10 min. Cook: 25 min.
Makes
12 servings (3/4 cup each)
Ingredients
- 3 pounds small red potatoes, quartered
- 1-pound fresh asparagus, trimmed and cut into 2-inch pieces
- 2 cups sliced radishes
- 6 green onions, sliced
- 2 tablespoons chopped fresh chives

2 tablespoons chopped fresh parsley
VINAIGRETTE:
- 3/4 cup olive oil
- 1/4 cup champagne vinegar or white vinegar
- 1 tablespoon Dijon mustard
- 1/2 teaspoon salt

1/4 teaspoon coarsely ground pepper
Directions

1. Place potatoes in a large saucepan; add water to cover. Bring to a boil. Reduce heat; cook, uncovered, 10-15 minutes or until tender. Remove potatoes with a slotted spoon; cool. Return water to a boil. Add asparagus; cook, uncovered, 2-3 minutes or just until crisp-tender. Remove asparagus and immediately drop into ice water. Drain and pat dry.
2. Transfer potatoes and asparagus to a large bowl; add radishes, green onions and herbs. In a small bowl, whisk vinaigrette ingredients until blended. Pour over potato mixture; toss gently to coat. Serve at room temperature or chilled. Stir before serving.

Nutrition Facts
3/4 cup: 213 calories, 14g fat (2g saturated fat), 0 cholesterol, 147mg sodium, 20g carbohydrate (2g sugars, 3g fiber), 3g protein. Diabetic Exchanges: 3 fat, 1 starch.

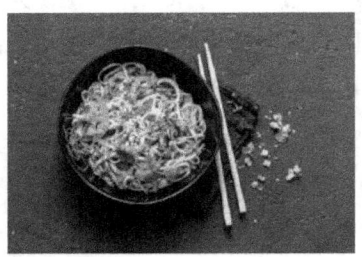

Vegetarian Pad Thai

Total Time
Prep/Total Time: 30 min.
Makes
4 servings
Ingredients
- 6 ounces uncooked thick rice noodles
- 2 tablespoons packed brown sugar
- 3 tablespoons reduced-sodium soy sauce
- 4 teaspoons rice vinegar
- 2 teaspoons lime juice
- 2 teaspoons olive oil
- 3 medium carrots, shredded
- 1 medium sweet red pepper, cut into thin strips
- 4 green onions, chopped
- 3 garlic cloves, minced
- 4 large eggs, lightly beaten
- 2 cups bean sprouts
- 1/3 cup chopped fresh cilantro
- Chopped peanuts, optional

Lime wedges

Directions
1. Prepare noodles according to package directions. Drain; rinse well and drain again. In a small bowl, mix together brown sugar, soy sauce, vinegar and lime juice.
2. In a large nonstick skillet, heat oil over medium-high heat; stir-fry carrots and pepper until crisp-tender, 3-4 minutes. Add green onions and garlic; cook and stir 2 minutes. Remove from pan.
3. Reduce heat to medium. Pour eggs into same pan; cook and stir until no liquid egg remains. Stir in carrot mixture, noodles and sauce mixture; heat through. Add bean sprouts; toss to combine. Top with cilantro and, if desired, peanuts. Serve with lime wedges.

Nutrition Facts
1-1/4 cups: 339 calories, 8g fat (2g saturated fat), 186mg cholesterol, 701mg sodium, 55g carbohydrate (15g sugars, 4g fiber), 12g protein.

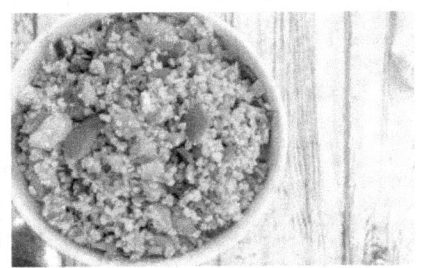

Mediterranean Bulgur Salad

Total Time
Prep: 15 min. Cook: 20 min. + cooling
Makes
9 servings
Ingredients
- 3 cups vegetable broth
- 1-1/2 cups uncooked bulgur
- 6 tablespoons olive oil
- 2 tablespoons lemon juice
- 2 tablespoons minced fresh parsley
- 1/2 teaspoon salt
- 1/4 teaspoon pepper
- 1 can (15 ounces) garbanzo beans or chickpeas, rinsed and drained
- 2 cups halved cherry tomatoes
- 1 cup chopped cucumber
- 8 green onions, sliced
- 1 package (4 ounces) crumbled feta cheese

1/2 cup pine nuts, toasted

Directions
1. In a large saucepan, bring broth and bulgur to a boil over high heat. Reduce heat; cover and simmer for 20 minutes or until tender and broth is almost absorbed. Remove from the heat; let stand at room temperature, uncovered, until broth is absorbed.
2. In a small bowl, whisk the oil, lemon juice, parsley, salt and pepper.
3. In a large serving bowl, combine the bulgur, beans, tomatoes, cucumber and onions. Drizzle with dressing; toss to coat. Sprinkle with cheese and pine nuts.

Nutrition Facts
1 cup: 298 calories, 17g fat (3g saturated fat), 7mg cholesterol, 657mg sodium, 31g carbohydrate (4g sugars, 8g fiber), 10g protein.

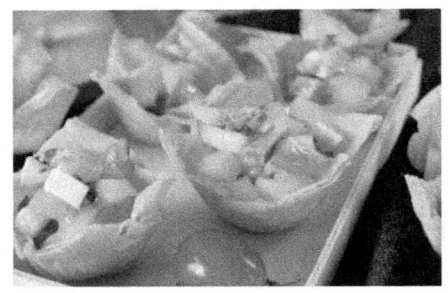

Veggie Quiche Bundles

Total Time
Prep: 25 min. Bake: 20 min.
Makes
1 dozen
Ingredients
- 1 cup chopped fresh mushrooms
- 1/2 cup diced zucchini
- 1/4 cup chopped red onion
- 1 tablespoon plus 1/3 cup butter, divided
- 1 plum tomato, seeded and diced
- 3 eggs
- 1/2 cup milk
- 1 tablespoon prepared pesto
- 1/4 teaspoon coarsely ground pepper
- 1/2 cup crumbled feta cheese
- 1/2 cup shredded part-skim mozzarella cheese

12 sheets phyllo dough (14 inches x 9 inches)

Directions

1. In a small skillet, saute the mushrooms, zucchini and onion in 1 tablespoon butter until mushrooms are tender; stir in tomato. In a small bowl, whisk the eggs, milk, pesto and pepper. In another bowl, combine feta and mozzarella cheeses.
2. Melt the remaining butter. Place one sheet of phyllo dough on a work surface; brush with butter. Repeat with three more sheets of phyllo, brushing each layer. Cut phyllo in half widthwise, then cut in half lengthwise. (Keep remaining phyllo covered with plastic wrap and a damp towel to prevent it from drying out.)
3. Repeat with remaining phyllo dough and butter (or vegan replacement). Carefully place each stack in a greased muffin cup. Fill each with 4 teaspoons vegetable mixture, 1 tablespoon cheese mixture and 4 teaspoons egg mixture. Pinch corners of phyllo together and twist to seal.
4. Bake at 325° for 20-25 minutes or until golden brown. Serve warm. Refrigerate leftovers.

Nutrition Facts
1 each: 141 calories, 10g fat (5g saturated fat), 75mg cholesterol, 188mg sodium, 8g carbohydrate (2g sugars, 1g fiber), 5g protein.

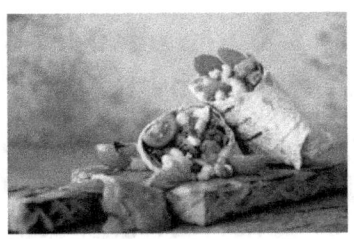

Lentil Taco Cups

Total Time
Prep: 25 min. Bake: 15 min.
Makes
6 servings
Ingredients
- 12 mini flour tortillas
- 1 can (15 ounces) lentils, drained
- 3/4 cup pico de gallo
- 1/2 cup enchilada sauce
- 2 tablespoons taco seasoning

2 cups shredded Mexican cheese blend, divided
CREMA:
- 1 cup sour cream
- 1/2 cup minced fresh cilantro
- 1 tablespoon lime juice
- 1/4 teaspoon sea salt

Shredded lettuce, sliced ripe olives and chopped tomatoes
Directions
1. Preheat oven to 425°. Press warm tortillas into 12 greased muffin cups, pleating sides as needed. In a large bowl, combine the lentils, pico de gallo, enchilada sauce and taco seasoning. Stir in 1-1/2

cups cheese. Divide lentil mixture among cups. Sprinkle with remaining cheese.
2. Bake until heated through and cheese is melted, 12-15 minutes. Meanwhile, for the crema, combine sour cream, cilantro, lime juice and sea salt. Serve cups with crema, lettuce, olives and tomatoes.

Tip
Skip the 1/2 cup cheese on top and switch to low-fat Greek yogurt to cut saturated fat by more than 50 percent.

Nutrition Facts
2 taco cups: 303 calories, 20g fat (11g saturated fat), 43mg cholesterol, 793mg sodium, 17g carbohydrate (3g sugars, 5g fiber), 14g protein.

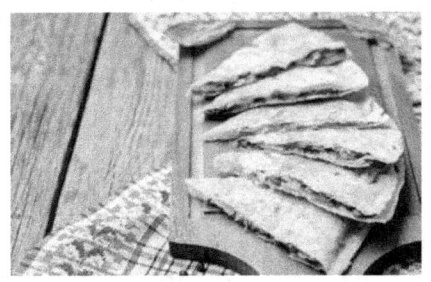

Grilled Feta Quesadillas

Total Time
Prep/Total Time: 20 min.
Makes
12 wedges
Ingredients
- 3 ounces fat-free cream cheese (or vegan replacement)
- 1/2 cup shredded reduced-fat Mexican cheese blend
- 1/3 cup crumbled feta cheese
- 1/2 teaspoon dried oregano
- 4 flour tortillas (6 inches), warmed
- 1/4 cup chopped pitted ripe olives
- 2 tablespoons diced pimientos

1 green onion, chopped

Directions
1. In a small bowl, beat cheeses with oregano until blended. Spread 3 tablespoons of cheese mixture over half of each tortilla; top with olives, pimientos and onion. Fold tortillas over.

2. Moisten a paper towel with cooking oil; using long-handled tongs, lightly coat the grill rack. Grill quesadillas, uncovered, over medium heat or broil 4 in. from the heat for 1-2 minutes on each side or until golden brown. Cut each quesadilla into three wedges. Serve warm.

Nutrition Facts
1 each: 62 calories, 3g fat (1g saturated fat), 6mg cholesterol, 198mg sodium, 5g carbohydrate (0 sugars, 0 fiber), 4g protein. Diabetic Exchanges: 1/2 starch, 1/2 fat.

Conclusion

Thank for making it through to the end of this book, let's hope it was filled with the right recipes for you and able to provide you with all of the tools you need to achieve your future meal prepping goals. Hopefully, you found some valuable recipes that you can add to your menu rotation or even some special ones that you can try out every now and then for a new taste. Either way, the goal of this book was to help you, so let's hope it did!

The next step is to keep sticking with your meal prep schedule and making sure to stay consistent with planning out and cooking your meals ahead of time. Don't forget that it always helps to change up your flavors so you don't get too bored or stuck in a rut, so try out something from this book or another source that might push you a little out of your comfort zone. You never know, you might end up enjoying the new experience!

Another step you can take in your meal prepping journey is to visit some other sources, maybe blogs or websites, that are filled with communities of other meal preppers who can help you on your way to diversifying your menu and staying consistent with your planning. Sometimes other people can be one of the best resources. And be sure to share all of the info that you learned from this book with any other meal preppers who might be interested!

www.ingramcontent.com/pod-product-compliance
Lightning Source LLC
Chambersburg PA
CBHW071437070526
44578CB00001B/118